Paediatric Data Interpretation

To the families and friends of those studying for exams

Paediatric Data Interpretation

John Walter, MRCP, DCH
Clinical Research Fellow
Institute of Child Health, University of London

Simon Lenton, MRCP, DRCOG
Lecturer in Community Child Health and Honorary Senior
Registrar in Paediatrics, Department of Child Health,
Southampton General Hospital

and

Cynthia M. Gabriel, FRCP, DCH
Consultant Paediatrician, St Albans City Hospital and
Queen Elizabeth II Hospital, Welwyn Garden City, Hertfordshire

Butterworths
London Boston Durban Singapore Sydney Toronto Wellington

All rights reserved. No part of this publication may be reproduced or transmitted in any form or by any means, including photocopying and recording, without the written permission of the copyright holder, application for which should be addressed to the Publishers. Such written permission must also be obtained before any part of this publication is stored in a retrieval system of any nature.

This book is sold subject to the Standard Conditions of Sale of Net Books and may not be re-sold in the UK below the net price given by the Publishers in their current price list.

First published, 1987

© **Butterworth & Co. (Publishers) Ltd, 1987**

British Library Cataloguing in Publication Data

Walter, John
   Paediatric data interpretation.
   1. Children—Diseases—Diagnosis—
   Problems, exercises, etc.
   I. Title II. Lenton, Simon III. Gabriel,
Cynthia M.
618.92'0075'076   RJ50

ISBN 0-407-00425-4

Library of Congress Cataloging-in-Publication Data

Walter, John (John Hugh)
   Paediatric data interpretation.

   Includes bibliographies.
   1.. Pediatrics--Examinations, questions, etc.
I. Lenton, Simon. II. Gabriel, Cynthia M.
III. Title. [DNLM: 1. Pediatrics--examination
questions. WS 18 W232p]
RJ48.2.W35   1987   618.92'0007'6   87-11661

ISBN 0-407-00425-4

Photoset by Butterworths Litho Preparation Department
Printed and bound in Great Britain by Anchor Brendon Ltd, Tiptree, Essex

Preface

Data interpretation is an important part of modern medical practice; it also forms one paper of the paediatric membership examination. Our aim in this book is two-fold: first to help those preparing for this examination, and secondly, we hope it will act as an aid in learning further paediatrics. To this end we have provided a discussion after each question and references for further reading, usually from the major paediatric textbooks.

We have tried to include a wide range of questions, although inevitably some subjects do not lend themselves to this format. The answers are those that we feel are the most appropriate for the history and data given, although there may be others that could be considered correct.

We have not included a chapter on normal data, as for this to be sufficiently comprehensive would have required too much space. Both Forfar and Arneil's and Nelson's textbooks on paediatrics included detailed sections on normal data. We would also recommend *Paediatric Chemical Pathology* by B. E. Clayton, P. Jenkins, and J. M. Round (1980) published by Blackwell Scientific Publications, Oxford.

We would like to thank the following for their help in the preparation of this book: Chris Wren, John Deanfield, Janet Drew, Gareth Morgan, the Departments of Neurophysiology in Southampton and at the Hospitals for Sick Children, Great Ormond Street, London, and the Department of Cytogenetics in Salisbury.

The standard texts referred to throughout in the answers are:

Nelson's Textbook of Pediatrics, 12th edn. (1983) edited by W. E. Nelson, R. E. Behrman and V. C. Vaughan. Philadelphia: W. B. Saunders

Forfar, J. O. and Arneil, G. C. (editors) (1985) *Textbook of Paediatrics*, 3rd edn. Edinburgh: Churchill Livingstone

Glossary

ALT (SGPT)	alanine transaminase
AST (SGOT)	aspartate transaminase
Cl INH	C1 esterase inhibitor
C3, C4	complements
ESR	erythrocyte sedimentation rate
FDP	fibrin degradation product
FEV_1	forced expiratory volume in 1 second
FVC	forced vital capacity
HLA	human lymphocyte antigen
hGH	human growth hormone
IVC	inferior vena cava
IVU	intravenous urogram
LH	luteinizing hormone
LHRH	luteinizing hormone releasing hormone
MCH	mean corpuscular haemoglobin
MCHC	mean corpuscular haemoglobin concentration
MCV	mean corpuscular volume
NBT	nitroblue tetrazolium
PCV	packed cell volume
PEFR	peak expiratory flow rate
PT	prothrombin time
PTTK	partial thromboplastin time (kaolin)
RBC	red blood cell count
TIBC	total iron-binding capacity
TLC	total lung capacity
TSH	thyroid stimulating hormone
TT	thrombin time
WBC	white blood cell count

Questions

Question 1

The ECG indicated on p.4 is from a 4-year-old boy.

Questions

(1) List three abnormalities.
(2) What is the diagnosis?

Question 2

A 9-year-old-girl presents with general lethargy, weakness and anorexia following her summer holiday 3 months earlier. Over the previous 2 days she had complained of abdominal pain and had vomited.
   On examination she is obviously suntanned, drowsy and lethargic; she is afebrile; her pubic development is Tanner stage 1.
   Initial investigation revealed:

Sodium	130 mmol/l
Potassium	5.8 mmol/l
Chloride	92 mmol/l
Urea	11 mmol/l
Glucose	2.9 mmol/l
Urine osmolality	380 mosmol/kg

Questions

(1) What additional physical sign should be sought?
(2) What is the diagnosis and how would you verify this?
(3) What is the likely cause?
(4) What is the initial management?
(5) What is the long-term management?

Question 3

A 5-year-old has been admitted with poor growth associated with loose stools.
   On examination his weight is below his height centile by two standard deviations. His liver is 3.5 cm below the right costal margin.
   The abnormalities present on the following investigations were consistent findings:

Hb	11.6 g/dl
WBC	4×10^9/l
neutrophils	14%
lymphocytes	78%
Bilirubin	17 µmol/l
AST (SGOT)	31 IU/l
ALT (SGPT)	28 IU/l
Alkaline phosphatase	400 IU/l

3

Question 1

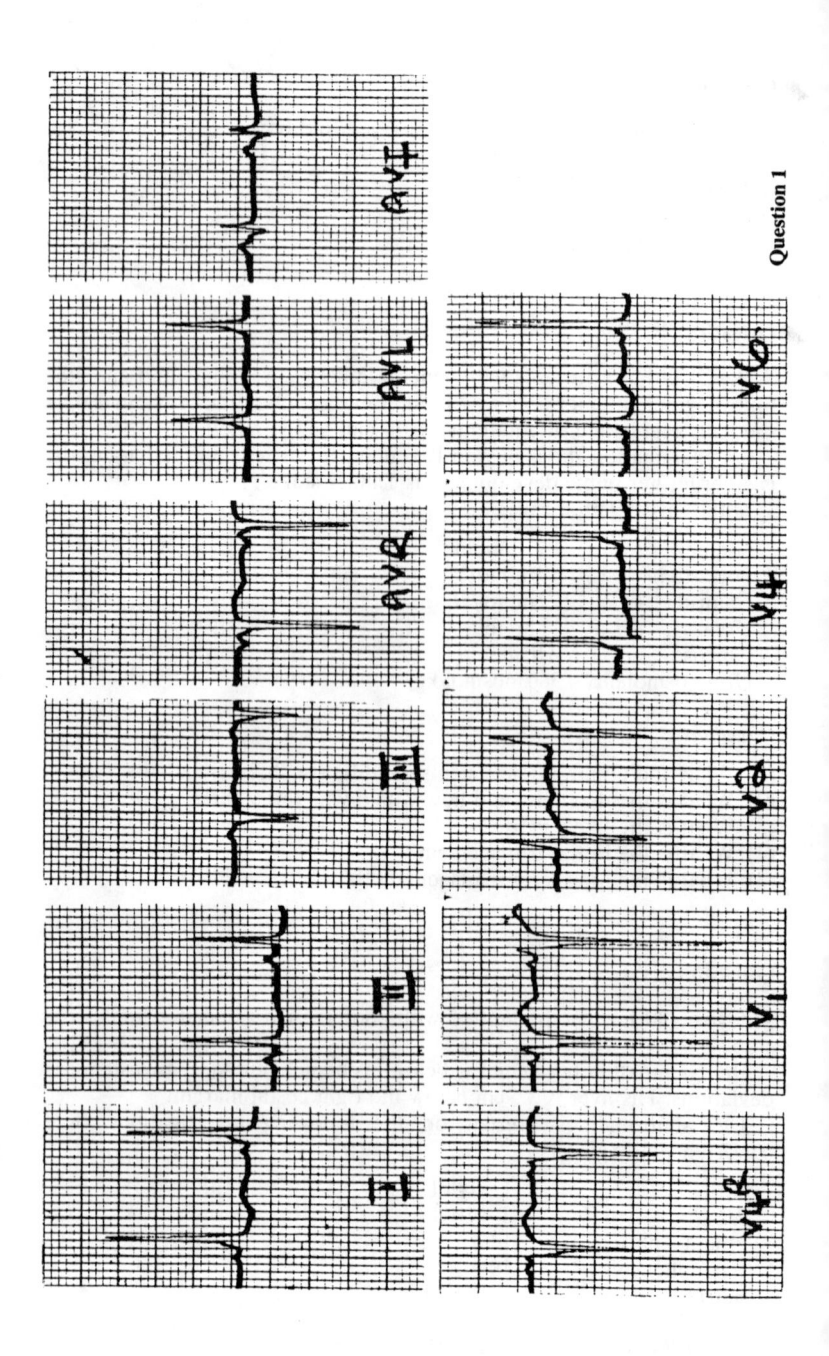

Sodium	140 mmol/l
Potassium	3.6 mmol/l
Urea	2.8 mmol/l
Bicarbonate	25 mmol/l

Questions

(1) What is the diagnosis?
(2) What are the next investigations?
(3) What is the management?

Question 4 ✓

A 13-month-old infant from West Africa presents with a 2-hour history of stridor not associated with fever.
Investigation reveals:

Hb	9.7 g/dl
WBC	13×10^9/l
neutrophils	60%
lymphocytes	38%
Sodium	135 mmol/l
Potassium	2.7 mmol/l
Urea	3.9 mmol/l
Calcium	1.7 mmol/l
Phosphate	0.5 mmol/l

Questions

(1) What is the cause of his stridor?
(2) What further investigations are needed to confirm the diagnosis?
(3) What is the first line in therapy?

Question 5 ✓

A 4-year-old boy is admitted to intensive care with septicaemia and hypotension.

Investigations

Plasma electrolytes:

Sodium	136 mmol/l
Potassium	4.9 mmol/l
Chloride	90 mmol/l
Bicarbonate	8 mmol/l
Glucose	5 mmol/l

$Na - (HCO_3 + Cl)$
$136 - 98 = 38$

Questions

(1) What further diagnosis is possible with these results?
(2) How would you confirm this?

Question 6 ✓

A 12-year-old boy is investigated after developing excessive bleeding following a dental extraction. His mother says she also 'bleeds easily'. On examination there was an extensive bruise over his right deltoid, no petechiae were present, and all joints had a full range of movements.
Results were as follows:

Hb 12.4 g/dl
WBC $8.7 \times 10^9/l$
Platelets $310 \times 10^9/l$
Prothrombin time (PT) 12.6 s (control 13.2 s)
Partial thromboplastin time (kaolin) (PTTK) 86 s (control 42.4 s)
Bleeding time 12 min

Questions

(1) What is the probable diagnosis?
(2) What investigation would confirm this?
(3) Why is the family history relevant?
(4) What advice would you give him and his parents?

Question 7 ✓

A 10-year-old girl is noted to have an enlarged spleen and icteric conjunctivae on routine school medical examination. She is otherwise well. There is no family history of note.

Investigations

Hb 10.2 g/dl
Blood film — spherocytes present
Serum bilirubin 50 µmol/l
Coombs' test negative
Bone marrow aspiration — erythroid hyperplasia
No blast cells seen

Questions

(1) What is the diagnosis?
(2) What further test would confirm this?

Question 8 ✓

A 3-year-old girl is investigated for steatorrhoea. Results were as follows:

Serum cholesterol 1.1 mmol/l
Serum triglyceride 0.13 mmol/l
Hb 12.9 g/dl
Blood film, acanthocytosis
Red cell peroxide haemolysis increased

Questions

(1) What is the diagnosis? AR
(2) How would you confirm this?
(3) What is the treatment?

Question 9 ✓

A 5-day-old breast-fed term infant weighing 3.85 kg who is feeding well is found to be jaundiced. Results so far are as follows:

Bilirubin	250 µmol/l
conjugated	31 µmol/l
Group A positive	
Coombs' negative	
Hb	14.5 g/dl
WBC	13.7 × 10⁹/l
ALT (SGPT)	27 IU/l
AST (SGOT)	29 IU/l
Alkaline phosphatase	210 IU/l
TSH	3 mU/l

Prolonged Jaundice
TORCH
Hep B
α₁ antitrypsin
aa screen
TFT's
Sweat Test

Questions

(1) What is the most likely cause of the jaundice?
(2) What else should be considered?
(3) How would you manage this baby?

Question 10 ✓

The following results were obtained at cardiac catheterization of an 18-month-old boy:

Site	Pressure (mmHg)	Oxygen saturation (%)
Superior vena cava		70
Right atrium	mean 8 ↑	72 ↑
Inferior vena cava		69
Right ventricle	60/0–8 ↑	89 ↑
Pulmonary artery	52/20, mean 32 ↑	91
Left atrium	mean 11	100
Left ventricle	90/0–11	100
Aorta	90/58, mean 75	100

Qp
Qs

Questions

(1) List two abnormalities present.
(2) What treatment is indicated?

Question 11 ✓

The medical paediatric team is asked to see a child of 3 years on the surgical ward who has just had a convulsion.

Two days before the child had a bowel resection for an intussusception which was not reducible and ischaemic at the time of operation.

Since the operation the child has received 110 ml/kg per day of 5% dextrose and has been apyrexial.

The electrolytes from this morning are:

Sodium	113 mmol/l
Potassium	3.1 mmol/l
Chloride	88 mmol/l
Bicarbonate	20 mmol/l
Urea	1.6 mmol/l
Glucose	6.2 mmol/l

Questions

(1) What is the osmolality of the serum?
(2) What is the most likely cause?
(3) What further investigation would you like to confirm the diagnosis?
(4) How would you manage the child?

Question 12 ✓

A 12-year-old complains of headaches. On examination she is found to have a blood pressure of 150/100. There are no other abnormal physical signs.

Investigations so far reveal:

Plasma
  sodium   141 mmol/l
  potassium   3.0 mmol/l
  bicarbonate 35.0 mmol/l
  urea   3.8 mmol/l
Urine
  albumin positive
  blood negative
  WBC 3/high power field
  culture negative
IVU normal
Plasma renin activity (PRA)   (normal = <7 pg/ml per h)
  high inferior vena cava   10.9 pg/ml per h
  low inferior vena cava   5.8 pg/ml per h
  right renal vein   14.7 pg/ml per h
  left renal vein   8.2 pg/ml per h
Urine catecholamines, normal

Questions

(1) What is the pathophysiological cause of her hypertension?
(2) What is the likely anatomical cause?
(3) What would be the next step in the investigation?

Question 13 ✓

A 10-year-old boy is investigated for anaemia, abdominal pain and short stature.

Results

Hb	9.1 g/dl
MCV	120 fl
Iron	16 µmol/l
TIBC	50 µmol/l
Vitamin B_{12}	60 ng/l
Serum folate	10 µg/l
Red cell folate	200 µg/l

Schilling test
    4% radiolabelled vitamin B_{12} excreted
    following 30 mg intrinsic factor, 5% excreted

Questions

(1) What do these results indicate?
(2) What is the likely diagnosis?

Question 14 ✓

Two abnormalities were noted on ultrasound at 16/40 gestation. As a result an amniocentesis was performed which produced the following:

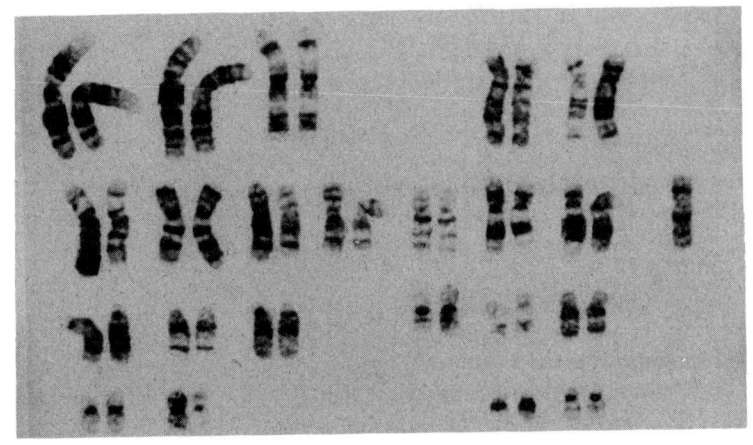

45 X0

Questions

(1) What is the diagnosis?
(2) What were the two abnormalities noted on ultrasound examination?

Question 15 ✓

A 13-year-old boy is investigated for short stature.
 On examination: height <3rd centile, weight 3rd centile; prepubertal.

Results

Bone age 10 years
TSH 3.0 mU/l
T_4 110 nmol/l
Insulin test

Time (min)	0	20	30	60	90	120
Glucose (mmol/l)	3.6	1.8	3.5	3.6	4.0	3.8
hGH (mIU/l)	5.5	6.0	7.9	12.9	12.5	10.0

Questions

(1) What is the most likely diagnosis?
(2) What further investigations would you advise?

Question 16 ✓

A 2-year-old boy with eczema is investigated for recurrent infections.

Hb	12.2 g/dl
WBC	4.5×10^9/l
neutrophils	90%
lymphocytes	10%
Platelets	40×10^9/l
IgG	110 IU/l (48–138)
IgA	160 IU/l (18–80)
IgM	10 IU/l (45–205)
IgE	600 IU/ml (1–222)

Low IgM

Questions
What is the most likely diagnosis?

Question 17 ✓

Questions

(1) Describe this EEG (*opposite*).
(2) Where is the likely lesion?
(3) Give two possible causes.

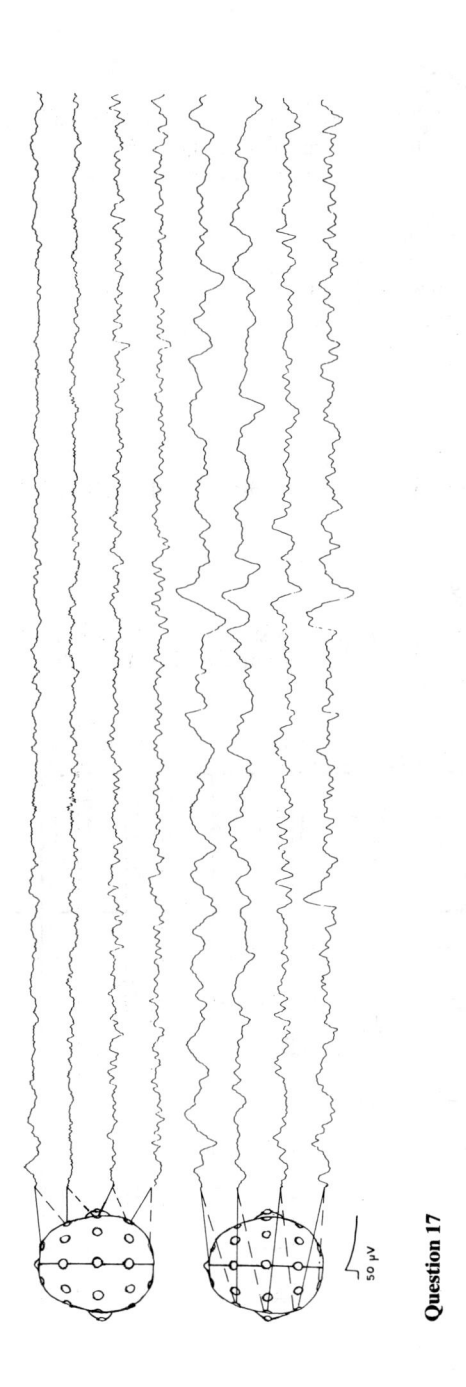

Question 17

Question 18

An 8-year-old girl suffers from recurrent epistaxes and easy bruising – at the age of two her sister seems to bruise easily also.
Investigation of the older girl reveals:

AR
1:4

Hb 11.6 g/dl
WBC 7.6×10^9/l
Platelets 360×10^9/l
Bleeding time 10.5 min
Prothrombin time normal
Partial thromboplastin time (PTT) normal
Factor VIII levels normal

Questions

(1) What is the diagnosis?
(2) Do you think her younger sister has the same disorder?

Question 19

A well child fails his hearing screening test and is referred for further investigations. The following audiogram was produced (right side only shown):

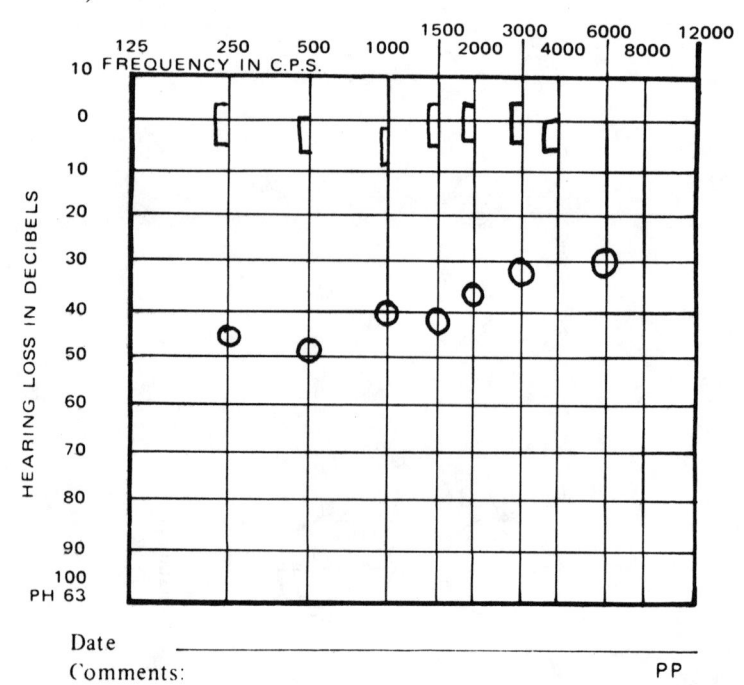

Date _____

Comments: PP

Questions

(1) What is shown in the audiogram?
(2) What type of hearing loss is shown?
(3) What is the likely cause of this?

Question 20 ✓

The ECG indicated on p.14 and cardiac catheter data are from a 7-year-old girl.

	Oxygen saturation (%)	Pressure (mmHg)
Superior vena cava	69	
Inferior vena cava	73	
Right atrium	88	mean 4
Right ventricle	92	40/3
Pulmonary artery	89	28/12
Left atrium	94	mean 5
Left ventricle	95	106/5
Right femoral artery	95	104/65

PS valve
grad. > 20

Questions

(1) What abnormalities are present on this ECG?
(2) What can you conclude from the catheter data?
(3) What is the probable diagnosis?

Question 21 ✓

A 4-year-old is admitted for investigation of polydipsia and polyuria. Initial electrolytes show:

Sodium   132 mmol/l
Potassium   3.7 mmol/l
Chloride   85 mmol/l
Calcium   2.3 mmol/l
Urea   2 mmol/l

Overnight water deprivation test urine osmolality: 685 mosmol/kg
Urinanalysis
  protein negative
  sugar   negative
  culture negative
  blood   negative

Questions

(1) Comment on these results.
(2) What conclusion would you come to?

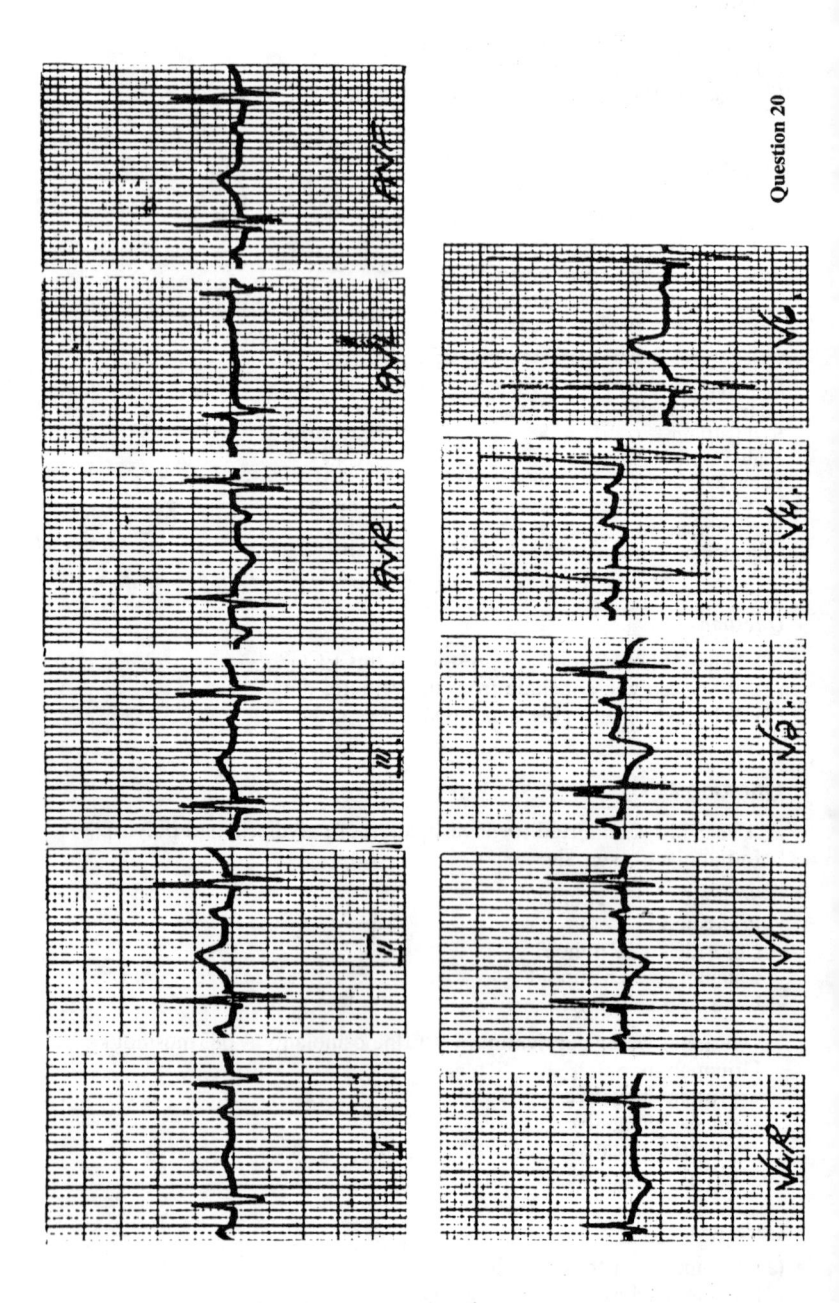

Question 20

Question 22 ✓

A 4-year-old boy is started on chemotherapy for newly diagnosed acute lymphoblastic leukaemia. Before treatment the serum creatinine was 55 mmol/l.
Routine biochemistry 3 days later shows:

Sodium	143 mmol/l
Potassium	8.1 mmol/l
Bicarbonate	9 mmol/l
Urea	45.3 mmol/l

Questions

(1) What abnormalities are shown?
(2) Why has this happened?
(3) What further investigation would you do?
(4) Could it have been prevented?

Question 23 ✓

On routine examination of urine in the outpatient department, a child was noted to be Clinitest positive.

Questions

(1) State four different types of substances other than glucose which will cause this.
(2) Name one further test for each substance.
(3) Which test is specific for glucose?

Question 24 ✓

A term infant becomes progressively jaundiced and at 14 days of age the results are as follows:

Serum bilirubin	270 μmol/l
direct	210 μmol/l
ALT (SGPT)	110 IU/l
AST (SGOT)	90 IU/l
Alkaline phosphatase	510 IU/l

Questions

(1) What form of hyperbilirubinaemia is this?
(2) Which two main diagnoses should be considered?
(3) Name two clinically important tests.

Question 25 ✓

A 2-year-old has been generally unwell for 9 days and on the day of admission developed a squint.
Cerebrospinal fluid (CSF) showed:

RBC $\quad\quad\quad\quad$ $29 \times 10^6/l$
WBC $\quad\quad\quad\quad$ $230 \times 10^6/l$
$\quad$ 50% lymphocytes
Protein $\quad\quad\quad$ 800 mg/l
Glucose $\quad\quad\:$ 1.7 mmol/l
(Plasma glucose 4.3)
Gram stain – no organism seen

Questions

(1) What is the probable diagnosis?
(2) What two further tests would you perform?
(3) What would your initial therapy consist of?

Question 26 ✓

A 7-day-old male infant, born at term, Apgar scores 8 at 5 min, 10 at 10 min, birth weight 3.6 kg, is seen because of poor feeding and lethargy.
On examination, weight is 3.1 kg, hypotonic, lethargic and clinically dehydrated; hyperpigmented scrotum.

Investigations

Hb $\quad\quad\quad\quad\quad\quad$ 20 g/dl
WBC $\quad\quad\quad\quad\:\:$ $25 \times 10^9/l$
Serum sodium $\quad\:\:$ 118 mmol/l
Serum potassium 5.3 mmol/l
Urinary sodium $\:\:$ 80 mmol/l

Questions

(1) What immediate treatment would you give?
(2) What is the most likely diagnosis?

Question 27 ✓

An 11-year-old boy who is breathless on exertion has the following lung function tests:

TLC $\quad$ 3250 ml
PEFR $\:$ 260 l/min
FVC $\:\:$ 2000 ml
FEV_1 $\:\:$ 1920 ml
Diffusion capacity: reduced

Questions
(1) What is the underlying physiological abnormality?
(2) Name five causes.   oedema
infiltrat
inflam / fibrosis

Question 28 ✓

A 5-month-old girl is admitted to hospital with severe diarrhoea and vomiting. On examination: pulse 160/min, BP 70/40, decreased skin turgor and dry mucous membranes.

Investigations
Plasma electrolytes
   sodium   125 mmol/l
   potassium 3.8 mmol/l
   urea   12 mmol/l
   creatinine 270 μmol/l
   calcium   2.3 mmol/l
Blood glucose 4 mmol/l
Urine
   sodium   4 mmol/l
   osmolality 580 mosmol/kg
   urea   258 mmol/l
Urine output approximately 0.6 ml/kg per h

125
·3.8
128.8
257.6
12
4
273.6

Questions
(1) What diagnosis can be made on the basis of the clinical findings and plasma electrolytes?
(2) What complication has arisen?

Question 29 ✓

A previously well 13-year-old girl presents with lethargy, pallor and difficulty concentrating at school.
On examination she has anterior and posterior cervical lymphadenopathy and axillary lymphadenopathy. She also has a degree of hepatosplenomegaly.
Investigations reveal:

Hb   7.4 g/dl
WBC   10.7 × 10^9/l
Reticulocytes 12%
Red cells described as being spherocytotic, anisocytotic and poikilocytic
Urine
   haemoglobin negative
   urobilinogen positive

Questions

(1) What type of anaemia has been described?
(2) Name three types of disease process which might present in this way.
(3) Suggest one useful investigation for each of the processes you have mentioned.

Question 30 ✓

The ECG indicated was taken from a 2-year-old girl following corrective surgery for tetralogy of Fallot.

Question

What abnormality is shown?

Question 31 ✓

A 12-month-old infant is investigated for severe failure to thrive. The pregnancy had been complicated by hydramnios and at birth she was noted to have abdominal distension. She required two exchange transfusions in the neonatal period. Diarrhoea had begun at 1 month of age and persisted ever since.

	Plasma (mmol/l)	Urine (mmol/l)	Stool (mmol/l)
Sodium	124	18	39
Potassium	1.3	24	26
Chloride	22	0	112
Bicarbonate	50	24	0
Urea	2.9	–	–
Creatinine	34	–	–

124 − 72

Questions

(1) What is the diagnosis?
(2) What is the treatment?

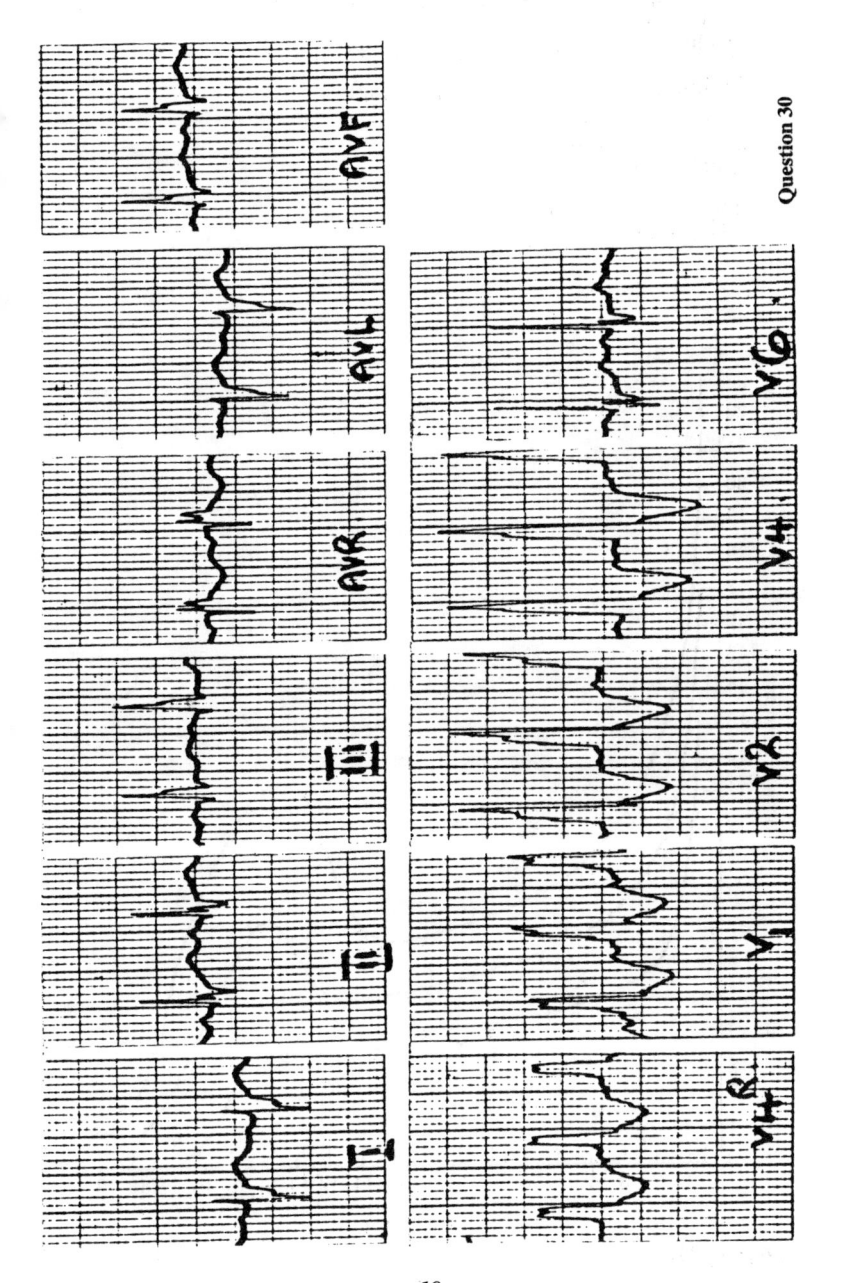

Question 30

Question 32

The following growth charts are from a 9-year-old boy, whose weight is on the 50th centile.

Results of investigations were as follows:

Skinfold thickness 7.5 mm (75th centile)
Bone age 5 years
Skull X-ray normal
Visual fields normal

Thyroxine 90 nmol/l
TSH 2.3 mU/l

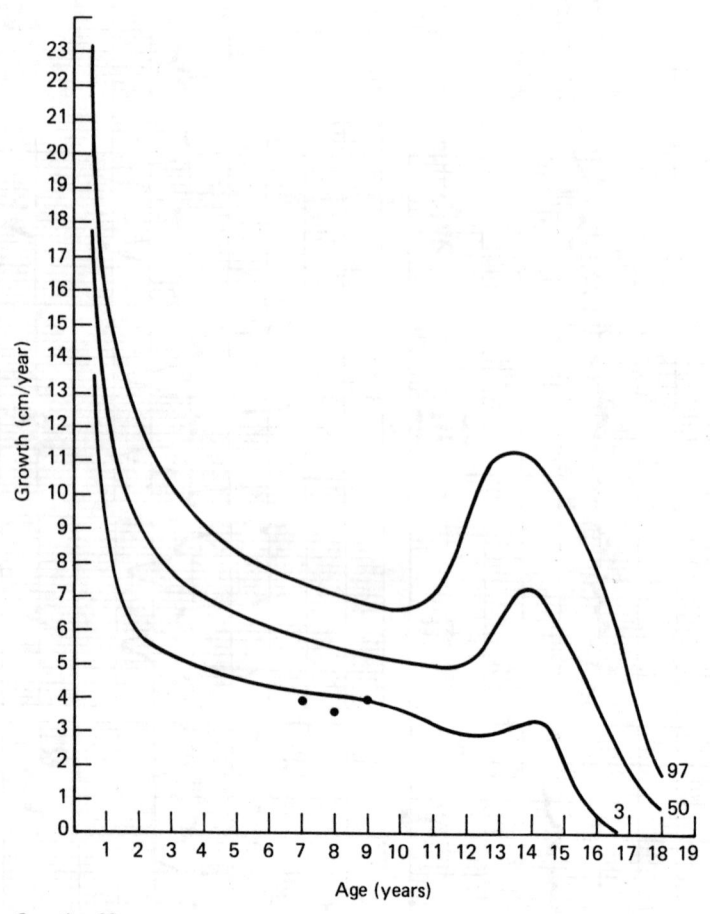

Question 32a

LHRH stimulation test
Time (min)	0	20	60
LH (U/l)	0.8	2.8	3.0
FSH (U/l)	0.5	2.6	3.2

Insulin test (0.1 U/kg)
Time (min)	0	20	30	60	90	120
Glucose (mmol/l)	3.5	1.7	2.9	3.2	3.3	3.4
Cortisol (nmol/l)	340	389	428	703	685	564
hGH (mIU/l)	4.0	4.7	6.1	5.8	4.3	4.4

Questions

(1) What is the diagnosis?
(2) What treatment is appropriate?

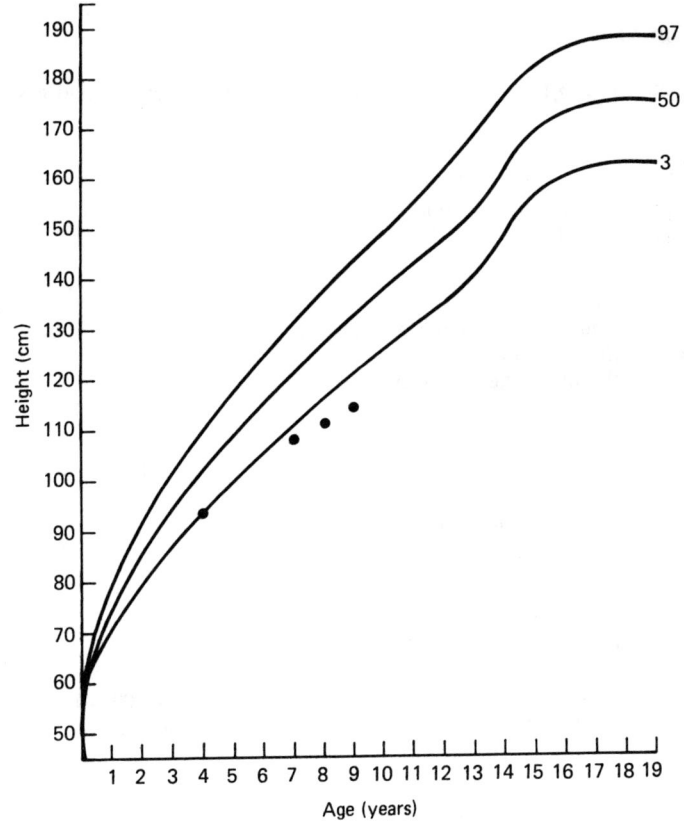

Question 32b

Question 33 ✓

A 15-year-old boy is investigated following an episode of renal colic.

Urine microscopy
  RBC $5000 \times 10^6/l$
  WBC $30 \times 10^6/l$
  No organisms seen
  Hexagonal crystals present
  IVU: bilateral radio-opaque calculi seen
  Urine cyanide–nitroprusside test: positive.

Questions

(1) What is the diagnosis?
(2) What would be found on urine amino acid chromatography?
(3) What treatment is required?

Question 34 ✓

A neonate in 72% headbox oxygen had the following arterial blood gas results:

  pH   7.05
  Pco_2 67 mmHg (8.9 kPa)
  Po_2 72 mmHg (9.6 kPa)
  Base excess   −10

Questions

(1) How do you account for the pH value?
(2) Explain the Po_2 value.
(3) What is the most likely diagnosis?

Question 35 ✓ $Pb < 1.4 \mu mol/l$

The following investigations are from a comatose 4-year-old boy:

  Hb   9.8 g/dl
  MCV   65 fl
  MCHC   28 g/dl
  Blood lead 5.7 μmol/l
  Urinary coproporphyrin 4 μmol/l (normal <0.15 μmol/l)
  Urinary porphobilinogen 0.1 mg/100 ml (normal <0.2 mg/100 ml)
  Urinary δ-aminolaevulinic acid 60 μmol/l (normal <39 μmol/l)

Questions

(1) Name three lines of treatment.
(2) What is the diagnosis?

Question 36 ✓

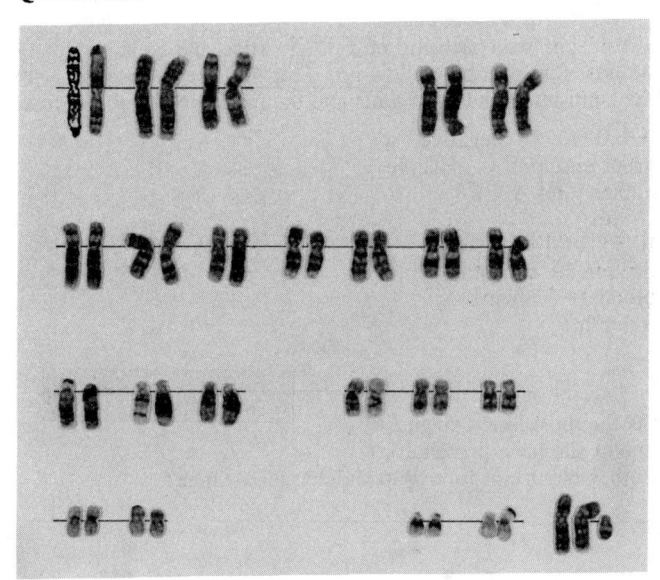

Questions

(1) Which clinical syndrome does this karyotype represent?
(2) What is the risk in the next pregnancy?   1 in 500
(3) What are the chances of the patient producing an affected child?

Question 37 ✓

A 10-year-old boy is admitted with acute asthma having been given an aminophylline suppository 45 minutes before.
  His arterial blood gases are:

pH	7.25
Pco_2	6.8 kPa (51 mmHg)
Po_2	6.2 kPa (47 mmHg)
Bicarbonate	18 mmol/l
Base excess	−4

Questions

(1) Give two possible causes for these figures.
(2) What would be the first two lines of management?

Question 38 ✓

An 11-year-old girl with arthritis of her left knee and right ankle for 8 years attends for routine follow-up. She has been treated with non-steroidal anti-inflammatory agents and the results in her notes show:

[handwritten left margin: Type I pauciar.]

Rheumatoid factor – negative
Antinuclear antibodies – positive
HLA studies – HLA-DR8
Hb 10.5 g/dl
WBC 10.5×10^9/l
Urine protein 2+ (Dipstik)
Urine blood 1+ (Dipstik)
ESR 35 mm/h

Questions

(1) What is the most likely diagnosis?
(2) Why might she have proteinuria?
(3) What other important follow-up should you arrange?

Question 39 ✓

The following is the constitution of a new locally produced baby formula recommended for infants from term to 3 months. You are asked to endorse this new product (values per 100 ml)

✗ Calories   110 g
  Protein   3.3 g
  Fat   3.7 g
  Sodium   52 mg (23 mmol/l)
  Potassium   140 mg (36 mmol/l)
  Calcium   120 mg (30 mmol/l)
  Phosphorus   98 mg (32 mmol/l)

Questions

(1) Suggest three changes to this formula.
(2) Name two clinical conditions that might result by feeding an infant this formula.
(3) What is this formula?
  [handwritten: C Milk + sugar]

Question 40 ✓

What abnormality is present on this ECG tracing from a 5-year-old girl?

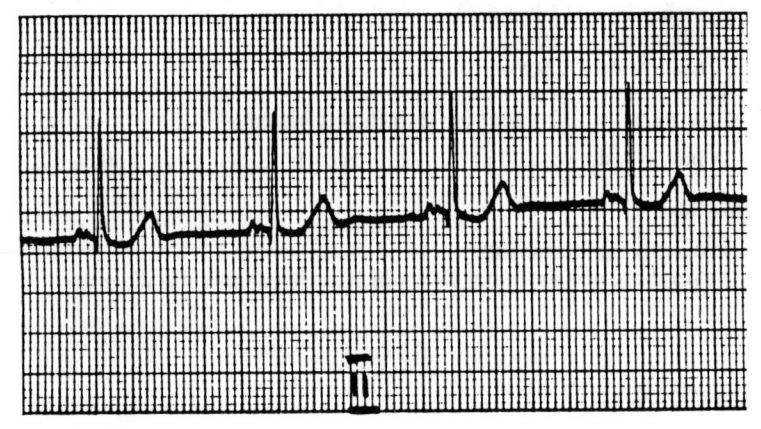

Question 40

Question 41 ✓

A 3-year-old boy with polydipsia and polyuria for 6 weeks is found to have glycosuria and blood sugar of 23.8 mmol/l. He is treated with neutral insulin (human, crb) but this is stopped after 3 weeks. Two weeks after stopping insulin he appears well and the following results were obtained:

Sodium 139 mmol/l
Potassium 4.1 mmol/l
Urea 3.5 mmol/l
Blood glucose (random) 3.9 mmol/l
Urine
  trace protein
  no glucosuria present

Question
What was the cause of the hyperglycaemia?

Question 42 ✓

A 2-day-old male infant, born at 36 weeks gestation, birth weight 2.05 kg, develops generalized oedema.

Investigations

Plasma
  sodium 128 mmol/l
  potassium 4.1 mmol/l
  bicarbonate 19 mmol/l

urea   5.8 mmol/l
albumin   10 g/dl
total protein 30 g/dl
Urine
protein   2.8 g/m² per 24 h (highly selective)

A previous sibling died at 3 weeks of age with oedema and septicaemia.

Questions

(1) What is the diagnosis?
(2) Are there any antenatal tests which might support this diagnosis?

Question 43 ✓

A 14-and-a-half-year-old boy with recurrent abdominal pains presents with a 2-week history of vomiting.
Electrolytes show the following:

Sodium   138 mmol/l
Potassium   3.1 mmol/l
Bicarbonate   36 mmol/l
Creatinine   211 µmol/l

Questions

(1) Describe the biochemical finding.
(2) What is the likely cause?
(3) What two further investigations should you consider?

Question 44 ✓

A 6-year-old girl has been noted to become increasingly pale over the previous month. Prior to this she had no serious illnesses. On examination she is not dysmorphic, has a resting tachycardia and a soft systolic flow murmur at the left sternal edge. She has some shin bruising. There is no organomegaly.
Investigation shows:

Hb   6.9 g/dl
WBC 1.2×10^9/l
Platelets 20×10^9/l
Reticulocytes <1%

Questions

(1) What has been described?
(2) Suggest two causes in this girl.

Question 45 ✓

A 3-year-old girl has bilateral breast development and irregular vaginal bleeding.
   On examination, her height is >97th centile; no cutaneous lesions; a large uterus and large left ovary palpable on rectal examination.

Investigations
   Bone age 5 years
   Skull X-ray normal
   Serum oestradiol 140 pmol/l (normal <50)

Questions
(1) What is the most likely diagnosis?
(2) What investigations would you do to confirm this?
(3) What is the treatment?

Question 46 ✓

The following investigations are from a previously well 13-year-old girl admitted to casualty unconscious.

   Arterial blood gases
      pH   7.3
      P_{CO_2} 3.3 kPa (25 mmHg)
      P_{O_2} 10.1 kPa (76 mmHg)
      Base excess −14
   Urine
      Clinistix negative
      Clinitest positive

Questions
(1) What is the likely diagnosis?
(2) What investigation would confirm this?

Question 47

A 12-hour-old term, breast-fed infant, birth weight 4.2 kg, has persistent small vomits containing blood. She appears otherwise well and there are no abnormal physical findings.
   Investigations are as follows:
   Hb   15.5 g/dl
   Platelets $240 \times 10^9/l$
   Prothrombin time   18 s; control 12 s
   Partial thromboplastin time (kaolin)   60 s; control 40 s
   Thrombin time   12 s; control 9 s
   Apt test   positive

Questions
(1) What is the diagnosis?
(2) What is the treatment?

Question 48

The following results are from a series of investigations on a 5- year-old boy. Normal values are shown in parentheses.

Serum immunoglobulins
   IgG   240 IU/ml (48–138)
   IgA   276 IU/ml (15–80)
   IgM   360 IU/ml (45–205)
Isohaemagglutinins : anti-B-titre   1:100 (1:5–1:640)
Phytohaemagglutinin (PHA) response normal
CH50   31 U/ml (20/40)
C3   1.2 g/dl (0.8–1.8)
C4   0.3 g/dl (0.22–0.8)
NBT dye reduction test: 0% positive cells.
In-vitro candida killing   reduced
In-vitro staphylococcal killing   reduced

Questions
(1) List five clinical problems that this boy might have.
(2) What is the diagnosis?
(3) What treatment is indicated for this disease?
(4) What is the inheritance?

Question 49

A 10-year-old is admitted for investigation of chest pain and breathlessness.
On examination he has dullness to percussion at the right base and chest X-ray shows a right pleural effusion.
A sample of fluid is taken and shows:

Specific gravity   1.028
WBC $9.5 \times 10^6/l$
   81% lymphocytes
Albumin   32 g/dl

Questions
(1) Which two diagnoses need to be considered?
(2) What further tests would you perform?

Question 50

Question
What abnormalities are present on this ECG?

Question 50

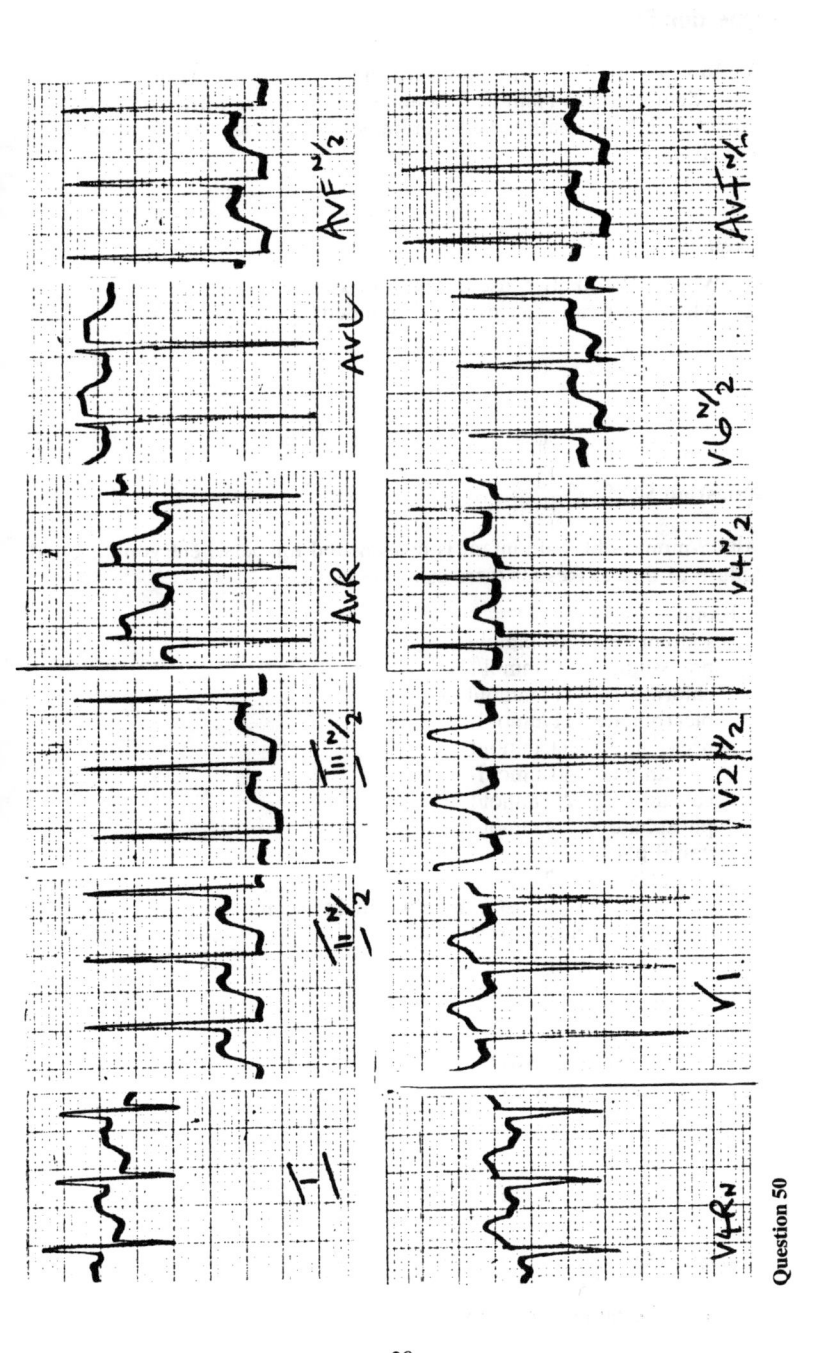

Question 51

A 16-year-old boy with long-standing, poorly controlled, insulin-dependent diabetes mellitus is below the 3rd centile for both height and weight. On examination he is prepubertal and has moderate hepatomegaly.

Questions

(1) What is the likely cause of his short stature?
(2) What other cause needs to be excluded?

Question 52

An 18-month-old male infant is investigated for persistent vomiting and failure to thrive. Results were as follows:

Blood
   sodium   133 mmol/l
   potassium   3.0 mmol/l
   chloride   112 mmol/l
   bicarbonate 11 mmol/l
   urea   3.0 mmol/l
   creatinine   40 mmol/l
   calcium   2.3 mmol/l
   phosphate 1.4 mmol/l
Arterial pH   7.18
Urine pH   5.2
Urinanalysis on Multistix: no abnormality seen
Urine amino acids: normal

Questions

(1) What is the diagnosis?
(2) What treatment is required?

Question 53

Consider the family tree shown.

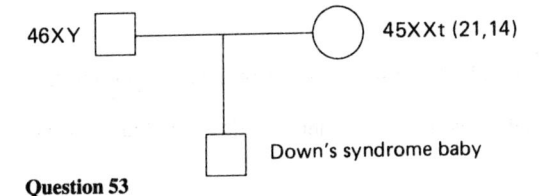

46XY ☐─────○ 45XXt (21,14)

☐ Down's syndrome baby

Question 53

Questions

(1) What is the genotype of the son?
(2) What are the chances of a further Down's syndrome child for these parents?

Question 54 ✓

A 2-month-old male infant with hepatomegaly is investigated for prolonged jaundice.
  Investigation results:

Serum bilirubin   205 µmol/l
  conjugated bilirubin 190 µmol/l
AST (SGOT)   400 U/l
ALT (SGPT)   280 U/l
Urinary reducing substances negative
^{99m}Tc-labelled HIDA isotope liver scan: isotope excreted into small bowel
Septic screen: negative on two separate occasions
Torch screen: negative
Liver biopsy: giant cell hepatitis
α_1-Antitrypsin phenotype: PiZZ
Thyroid function normal

Questions

(1) What is the likely cause of this child's hepatitis?
(2) What other problems may occur with this disease in later life?

Question 55 ✓

A 6-year-old boy with splenomegaly is investigated for anaemia.

Results

Hb	5.2 g/dl
MCV	65 fl
Serum iron	20 µmol/l
HbA	undetectable
HbS	65%
HbF	35%

Questions

(1) What is the diagnosis?
(2) What is haemoglobin electrophoresis of the parents' blood likely to show?
(3) What factors should be considered when deciding whether splenectomy is indicated?

Question 56

A 1-year-old boy has diarrhoea and vomiting. On examination he is extremely irritable, has cool peripheries and a blood pressure of 68/40.
Initial investigations:

Plasma
    sodium   162 mmol/l
    potassium   4.4 mmol/l
    bicarbonate   17 mmol/l
    urea   11.6 mmol/l
    glucose   4.3 mmol/l

Questions

(1) What is the diagnosis?
(2) What fluid regime would be appropriate for treating this boy?

Question 57

A pale 6-month-old Asian baby, who is otherwise well, has the following full blood count:

Hb   10.1 g/dl
WBC 7.0×10^9/l
MCV   79 fl
MCH   25 pg
MCHC   31 g/dl
HbA_2 1.3%
HbF   1%

Questions

(1) Comment on these parameters.
(2) What treatment would you prescribe?

Question 58 ✓

A child does the following drawing of 'Mummy':

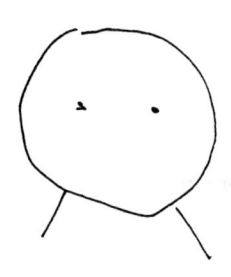

and copies a ladder:

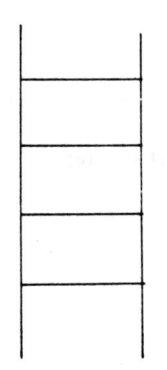

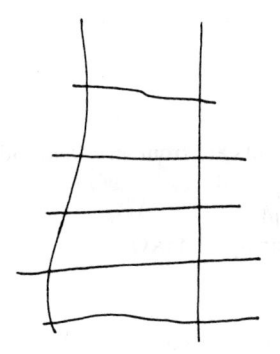

Question

How old is the child?

Question 59 ✓

A 5-year-old girl has early breast and pubic hair development. Her mother had noticed blood staining on her underwear on several occasions over the last 3 years.

On examination her height is 123 cm (>97th centile), weight 24 kg (90th centile), breast and pubic hair stage II. One café-au-lait spot (6 × 7 cm) left upper thigh.

Investigations

    Bone age   10 years
    Plasma oestradiol 176 pmol/l

Questions

(1) What is the diagnosis?
(2) What further investigation would help to confirm this?

Question 60 ✓

Questions

(1) What abnormality is shown on this ECG tracing (opposite)?
(2) What treatment is required?

Question 61 ✓

The following results are from an 8-year-old girl with short stature:

    TSH 15 mU/l
    T_4 70 nmol/l
    Chromosome analysis: 45XO

Questions

(1) What is the cause of this child's short stature?
(2) What is the likely cause of her abnormal thyroid function?
(3) What investigation would confirm this?

Question 62 ✓

A 7-year-old boy is admitted to the ENT ward for nasal polypectomy having had a chronic cough and postnasal drip for many years.
    Preoperative blood gases were as follows:

    pH   7.38
    Pco_2 65 mmHg (8.6 kPa)
    Po_2 55 mmHg (7.3 kPa)
    Bicarbonate 31 mmol/l

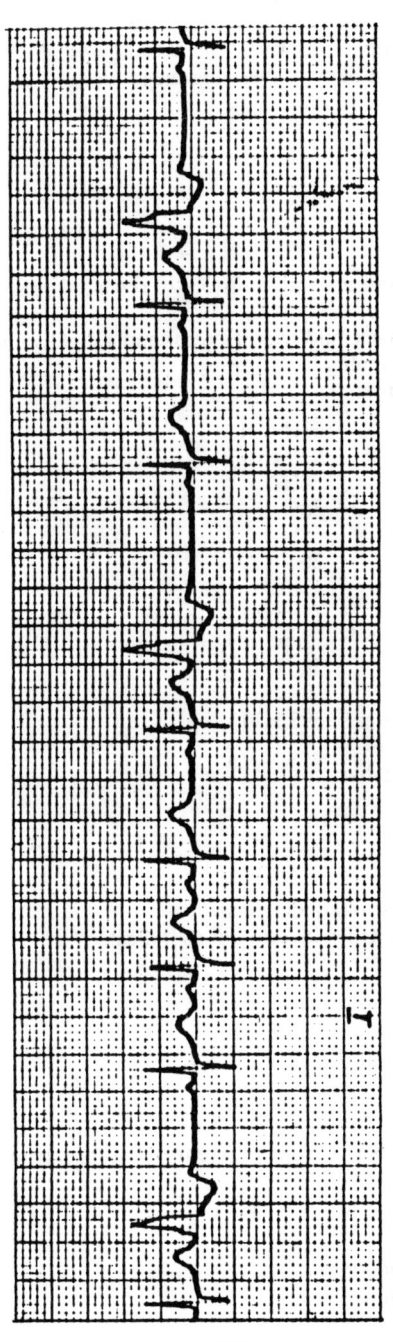

Question 60

Questions

(1) What abnormality is shown by the blood gases?
(2) What is the most likely underlying diagnosis?

Question 63

A 3-year-old girl presents with a history of repeated episodes of jaundice since one year of age.
Examination reveals mild scleral icterus and a slightly enlarged liver but otherwise no abnormality.
Investigation shows:

Hb	11.1 g/dl
WBC	9.3×10^9/l
neutrophils	54%
lymphocytes	38%
monocytes	6%
eosinophils	2%
Reticulocytes	1.4%
ESR	11 mm/h
Bilirubin	71 µmol/l
AST	58 IU/l
ALT	69 IU/l
Alkaline phosphatase	595 IU/l

Urine: bile +++
Urobilinogen negative

Questions

(1) What is the most likely diagnosis?
(2) Are there any further investigations indicated?

Question 64

The audiogram shown is from a 5-year-old whose tympanometry was normal.

Questions

(1) Describe the audiogram.
(2) Name two common causes.

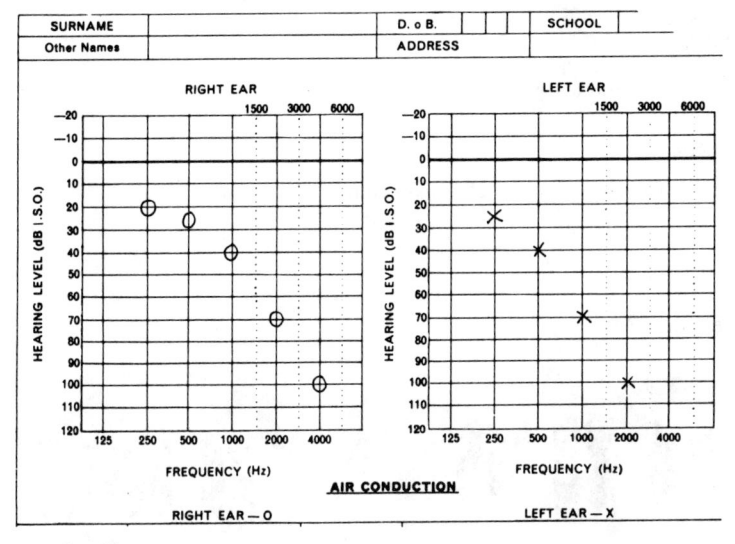

Question 64

Question 65

A 5-month-old bottle-fed girl is investigated for weight loss, vomiting, constipation and developmental delay. On examination she is irritable, hypotonic and has a systolic murmur.

Results

Calcium	3.6 mmol/l
Phosphate	1.32 mmol/l
Alkaline phosphatase	170 U/l

Questions

(1) What is the most likely diagnosis?
(2) What is the treatment?

Question 66

The following results are from an 8-year-old boy.

Hb	6.5 g/dl
WBC	7×10^9/l
RBC	4.0×10^{12}/l

PCV   23.5%
MCV   58 fl
MCHC   28 g/dl
Platelets $200 \times 10^9/l$

Question

Give four possible causes of his anaemia.

Question 67 ✓

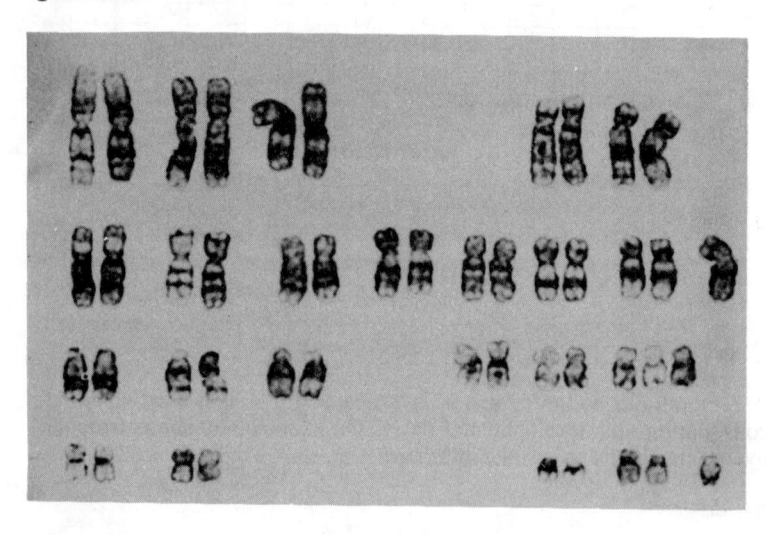

Questions

(1) What is the diagnosis?
(2) What hand abnormality is likely to be present?

Question 68 ✓

The following are complement assay results from a 13-year-old girl suffering from recurrent attacks of urticaria and colicky abdominal pain.

CH50   29 units/ml (20–40)
C3   1.0 g/dl (0.8–1.8 g/dl)
C4   0.4 g/dl (0.2–0.8 g/dl)
C1 INH   0.3 g/dl (1.5–3.0 g/dl)

Questions

(1) What is the diagnosis?
(2) What treatment is available?
(3) Name one serious complication.

Question 69

An 11-year-old Thai girl has recurrent abdominal pain and diarrhoea, diagnosed as Crohn's disease. As a result she is started on sulphasalazine on a regular basis.

She returns to outpatients in 2 months complaining of feeling weak and having no energy.

Her routine urine analysis shows 1+ blood and on examination she is slightly jaundiced with a pyrexia of 38°C.

Questions

(1) What is the cause of the blood in her urine?
(2) Is this related to the jaundice?
(3) What single test would be most useful here?

Question 70

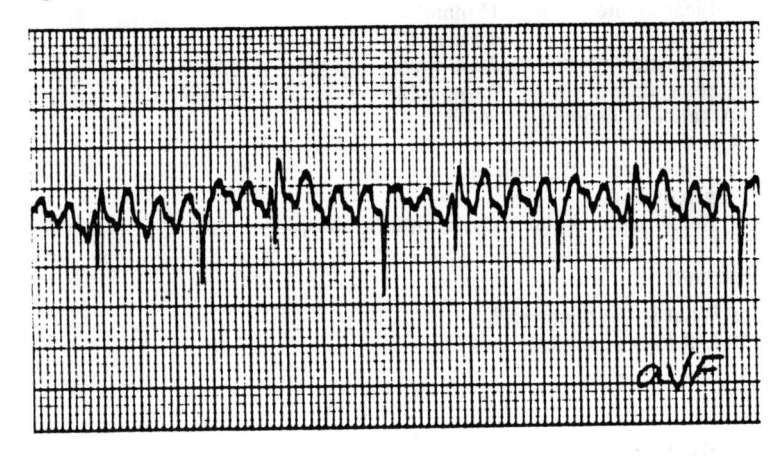

Questions

(1) What abnormality is present on this ECG?
(2) What treatment would you consider?

Question 71

An 11-year-old boy with diabetes mellitus and sensorineural deafness develops polyuria and polydipsia despite apparently good diabetic control.
Water deprivation test:

Weight loss approx. 5% body weight
Maximum urine osmolality   80 mosmol/kg
Maximum plasma osmolality   307 mosmol/kg
Urine osmolality following desmopressin intranasally   350 mosmol/kg

Questions

(1) What can you conclude from the results of the water deprivation test?
(2) What other abnormality might you expect to find?
(3) What is the diagnosis?

Question 72

The following results are from an 8-month-old infant with failure to thrive and radiological evidence of rickets.

Plasma electrolytes
   sodium   135 mmol/l
   potassium   3.2 mmol/l
   chloride   115 mmol/l
   bicarbonate   15 mmol/l
   urea   4.5 mmol/l
   chloride *calcium*   2.2 mmol/l
   phosphate   0.6 mmol/l
Alkaline phosphatase   360 IU/l
Urine
   generalized aminoaciduria
   glycosuria
   percentage tubular reabsorption of phosphate   29%

Questions

(1) What is the diagnosis?
(2) List four possible causes.

Question 73

An 11-year-old girl presents with fatigue and weakness particularly after sports at school.
  On examination a squint can be demonstrated. Her growth is within the normal centiles for her age.

Spirometry following exercise shows:
FEV$_1$ 1000 ml
FVC   1200 ml
Blood gases

	Air	100% oxygen
pH	7.31	7.33
Pco$_2$	50 mmHg (6.7 kPa)	52 mmHg (6.9 kPa)
Po$_2$	55 mmHg (7.3 kPa)	190 mmHg (25.3 kPa)

Questions

(1) What do these results show?
(2) Which two tests would you next perform?
(3) What is the underlying diagnosis?

Question 74

A 24-hour-old male Chinese infant, born at 39 weeks gestation, has a serum bilirubin of 245 mmol/l. Further investigation results were as follows:

Hb 11.1 g/dl
Blood group O, Rh negative
Direct Coombs' test negative

Question
Give three possible diagnoses.

Question 75

An 8-year-old boy is noted to have become increasingly lethargic at school over the last few months. He now complains of pain in his legs during PE lessons.
On examination he looks pale and complains of pain at the limits of movement in his knees and wrists.
Biochemistry reveals:

Sodium   137 mmol/l
Potassium   5.8 mmol/l
Creatinine   450 μmol/l
Calcium   1.9 mmol/l
Phosphate   2.1 mmol/l
Alkaline phosphatase 1200 IU/l

Questions

(1) What is the cause of his leg pains?
(2) What is the underlying problem?
(3) What three further pieces of information are required to help in his acute management?

Question 76

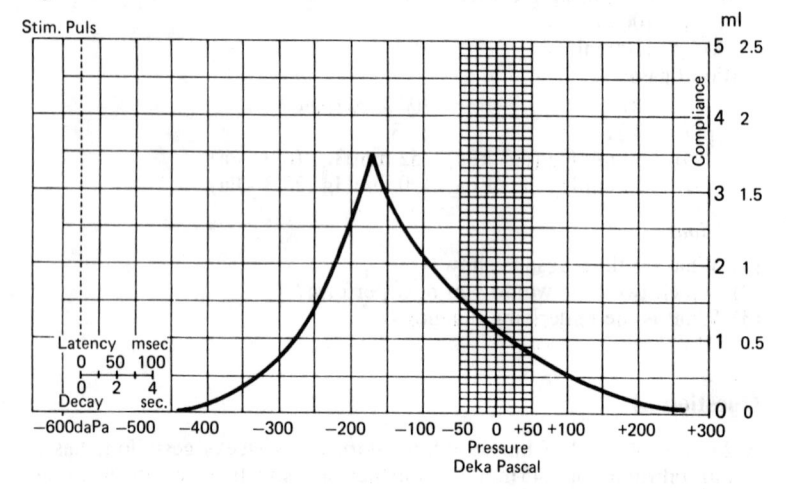

Examine the tympanogram above.

Questions

(1) Would you expect this child's hearing to be normal?
(2) At what pressure is the tympanic membrane most compliant?
(3) What is the most likely explanation of the above findings?

Question 77

A child can copy a circle, a cross and a square but cannot copy a triangle or a diamond.

Question

How old is the child?

Question 78

A 13-year-old girl presents in casualty with chest pain and breathlessness. Her arterial blood gases in room air are as follows:

Po_2 86 mmHg (11.5 kPa)
Pco_2 19 mmHg (2.5 kPa)
Bicarbonate   20 mmol/l

Questions

(1) What do they show?
(2) What is the likely diagnosis?

Question 79

An infant is discovered to be glucose-6-phosphate dehydrogenase deficient. On testing the parents the following results are obtained:

Father normal
Mother slightly decreased levels

Question

What are the chances of glucose-6-phosphate dehydrogenase deficiency in children of this couple (1) if male, (2) if female?

Question 80

The following rhythm strip is from an asymptomatic 13-year-old boy.

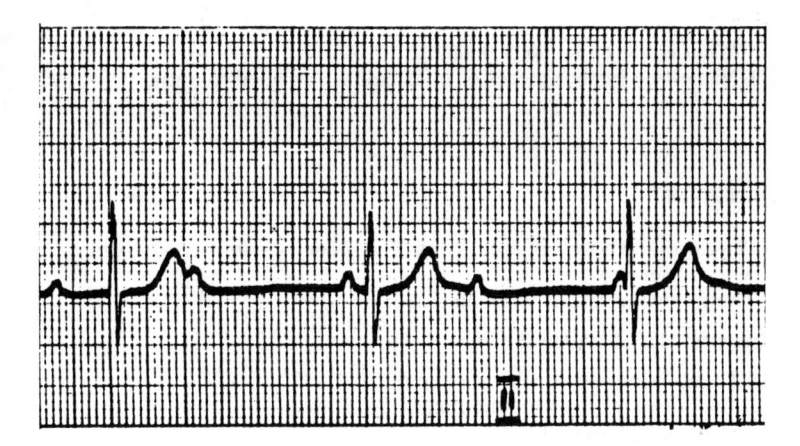

Questions

(1) What abnormality is present?
(2) What is the most likely aetiology?
(3) What treatment is required?

Question 81

An 8-year-old boy is admitted to hospital in an attempt to improve control of his diabetes. He has persistent morning glycosuria and ketonuria. He is presently on a total of 1.5 units of human insulin per kg per 24 hours.

Questions

(1) What is the most likely cause of the poor control?
(2) How would you change his treatment?

Question 82

A 9-year-old girl was taken to her GP with a 'flu'-like illness.
On examination she was jaundiced and her spleen was palpable (4 cm). Investigation showed:

Hb	9.5 g/dl
PCV	28%
RBC	$32 \times 10^{12}/l$
MCHC	30 g/dl
Bilirubin	33 µmol/l
Reticulocytes	6.9%

Coombs' test positive

Questions

(1) What is the most likely diagnosis?
(2) Name two further pieces of information you need to know.

Question 83

A 9-year-old whose epileptic control is poor is admitted following a prolonged seizure.
 The following results were obtained:

Phenytoin 48 (therapeutic range 40–80 µmol/l).

(1) Phenobarbitone 40 (therapeutic range 45–110 µmol/l)
(2) Primidone 21 (therapeutic range 25–55 µmol/l)
(3) Calcium 2.1 mmol/l
(4) Phosphate 1.4 mmol/l
(5) Alkaline phosphatase 600 IU/l (normal adult range 60–190 IU/l)
(6) Creatinine kinase 550 IU/l (normal <60 IU/l)

Question

Explain the values in (1)–(6).

Question 84

A baby is born at home to a 16-year-old mother. The baby weighed 2.4 kg at birth and had good Apgar scores.

The baby is transferred into hospital because the midwife is concerned about her slow feeding.

On examination the infant looks light for dates. The liver is 3 cm enlarged and the red reflexes seem hazy.

Over the next 3 days the baby starts to vomit and becomes noticeably jaundiced. Results are:

Total bilirubin	270 µmol/l
Sodium	143 mmol/l
Potassium	3.7 mmol/l
Bicarbonate	19 mmol/l
Urea	4.9 mmol/l
Hb	15.1 g/dl
WBC	8.9×10^9/l
Platelets	263×10^9/l

Questions

(1) What two diagnoses are possible?
(2) Name two tests.
(3) How would you manage this infant?

Question 85

A 10-year-old girl is admitted to hospital following a focal convulsion. Investigations were as follows:

CSF cells
    RBC $11\,000 \times 10^6$/l
    WBC 180×10^6/l, 60% neutrophils
Glucose 3.8 mmol/l
Protein   0.9 g/l
Gram stain, no organisms seen
EEG: focal periodic slow wave abnormality over left temporal lobe

Questions

(1) What is the probable diagnosis?
(2) How might this be confirmed?
(3) What specific treatment should be given?

Question 86 ✓

A male infant aged 5 days, born at 36 weeks gestation, birth weight 4.3 kg, is investigated for persistent hypoglycaemia. Results are as follows:

Sodium	135 mmol/l
Potassium	3.8 mmol/l
Urea	3.7 mmol/l
Calcium	2.01 mmol/l
Blood sugar	1.4 mmol/l
Plasma insulin	18 mU/l

Question
Give three possible causes.

Question 87

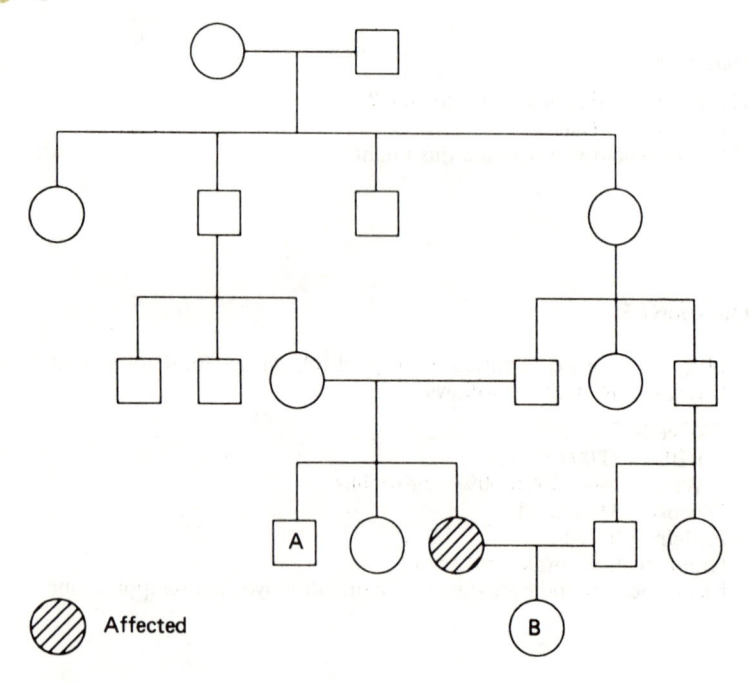

Questions
(1) What is the inheritance pattern shown?
(2) What are the chances of son A producing affected children if the

carriage rate in the general population is 1:35 (presuming he marries an unrelated person)?
(3) What are the risks of child B being affected?

Question 88

The EEG on p. 48 is from a 4-month-old infant.

Questions

(1) Describe the EEG abnormality.
(2) What is the likely clinical condition?
(3) What would you need to ask in the history?
(4) Name three additional tests.

Question 89

This DTPA (diethyltriamine pentaacetic acid) renogram was from a 9-year-old boy who had recurrent abdominal pains. On three occasions he had documented urinary tract infections.

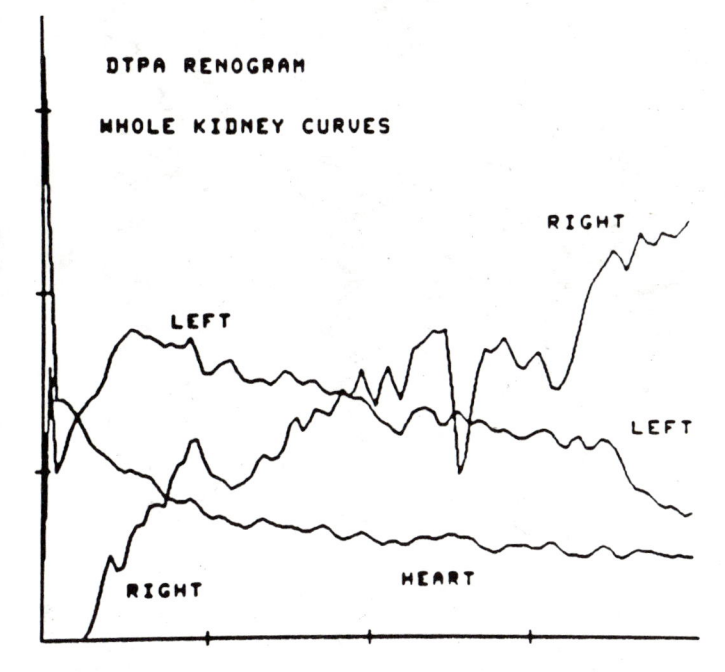

DTPA RENOGRAM

WHOLE KIDNEY CURVES

RIGHT

LEFT

LEFT

RIGHT

HEART

Questions

(1) What does it show?
(2) What pathological diagnosis is most likely?

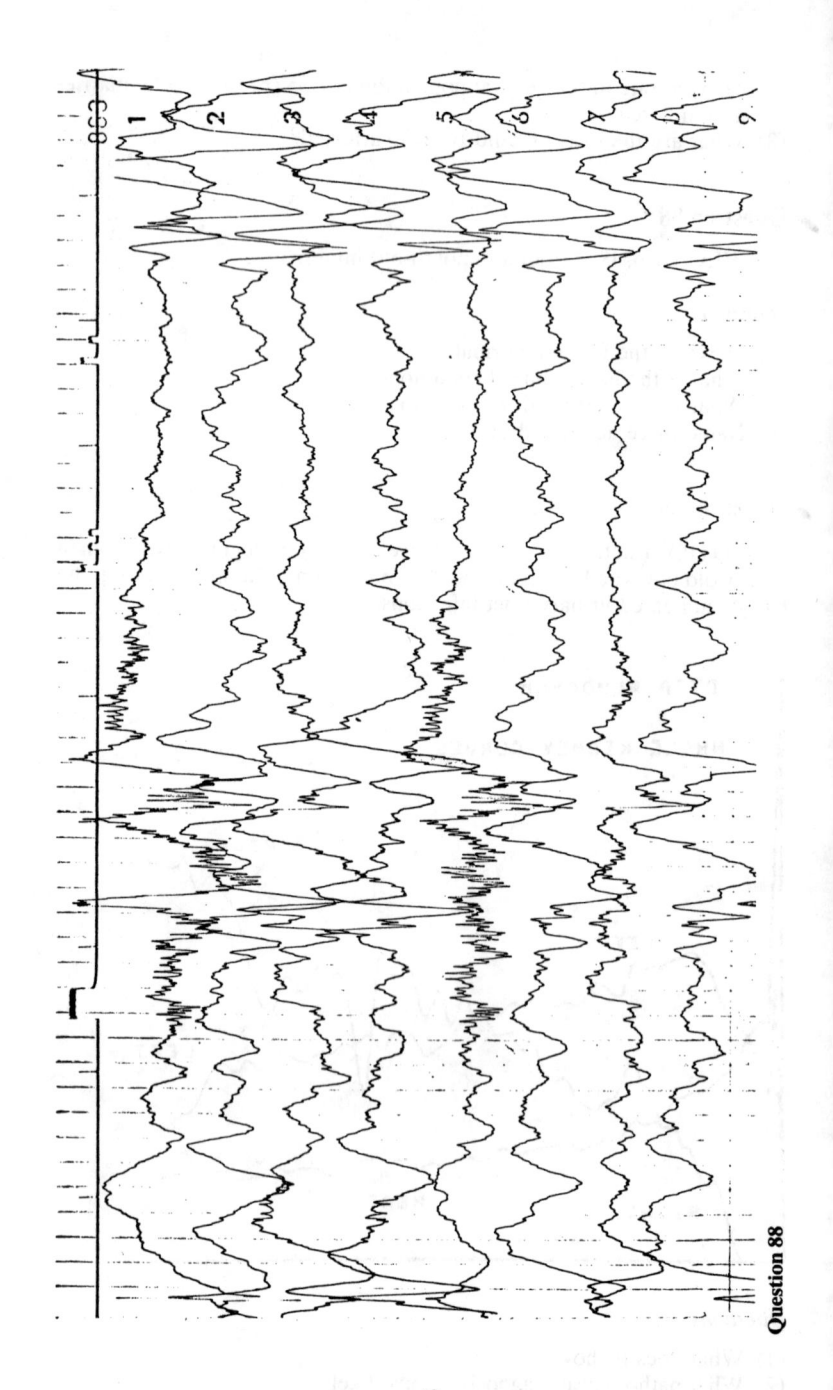

Question 88

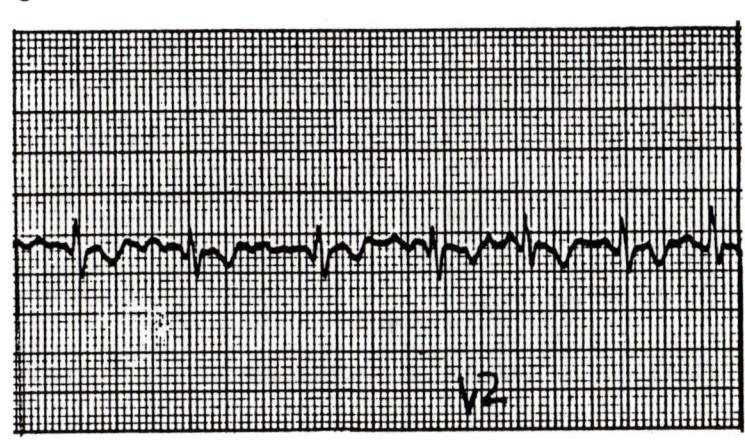

Question 90

Question
What abnormality is present on this ECG tracing?

Question 91

A 10-year-old boy was admitted to a surgical ward with abdominal pain. Investigations were as follows:

Hb	15.6 g/dl
WBC	$24 \times 10^9/l$
Sodium	125 mmol/l
Potassium	4.4 mmol/l
Urea	9.2 mmol/l
Serum osmolality	289 mosmol/kg

Questions
(1) What further simple investigations would you do?
(2) What is the likely diagnosis?

Question 92

A 7-year-old girl is investigated for polyuria and polydipsia.

Plasma electrolytes
sodium   141 mmol/l
potassium   3.2 mmol/l
bicarbonate 13 mmol/l
chloride   118 mmol/l
urea   5.8 mmol/l
calcium   2.3 mmol/l
blood glucose 3.2 mmol/l

Water deprivation test
weight loss 4.8% of body weight
urine osmolality 380 mosmol/kg

Plain abdominal X-ray: medullary nephrocalcinosis

Questions

(1) What is the diagnosis?
(2) What is the urine pH likely to be?
(3) What treatment is required?

Question 93

A child can name three colours, understands the prepositions 'under', 'on', 'behind' and comprehends hot and cold.
The child can sit unsupported but cannot be pulled to stand or walk.

Questions

(1) What is the minimum age of the child?
(2) Are there any comments to be made about this pattern of development?

Question 94

A 1-day-old premature infant of 29 weeks gestation, birth weight 1.8 kg, is given positive pressure ventilation for respiratory distress syndrome. He has marked bruising of the skin. Results of investigations were as follows:

Arterial blood gas
pH   7.25
Po_2 15 kPa (112.5 mmHg)
Pco_2 6.7 kPa (50 mmHg)
bicarbonate 15 mmol/l

Hb   13 g/dl
WBC 3×10^9/l
Platelets 80×10^9/l
Prothrombin time 15 s, control 12 s
Partial prothrombin time (kaolin) 90 s, control 40 s
Thrombin time 15 s, control 8 s
FDP   10 mg/dl
Sodium   134 mmol/l
Potassium   4.0 mmol/l
Urea   4.4 mmol/l

Questions

(1) What abnormalities are shown?
(2) What, if any, further investigations would you do?
(3) What three changes do you think are required in this baby's management?

Question 95

A 1-year-old boy has had frequent attacks of otitis media and pneumonia from the age of 4 months. His mother's brother also had recurrent bronchopneumonia and died in infancy.

Investigations

Hb   12.2 g/dl
WBC 7.2×10^9/l
   50% neutrophils
   45% lymphocytes
Sweat test: sweat sodium   15 mmol/l
IgG 14 IU/ml (40–122)
IgA   3 IU/ml (20–1100)
IgM 15 IU/ml (40–200)
Blood group B
Isohaemagglutinins not detected
Surface membrane immunoglobulins not detected
E-rosettes with sheep red blood cells 92% (normal 54–80%)
OKT3 92% (normal 49–63%)
Phytohaemagglutinin (PHA) response normal
NBT dye test: 99% NBT positive cells

Questions

(1) What is the most likely diagnosis?
(2) Why did symptoms only develop after 4 months of age?

Question 96

A 9-year-old girl, who had previously been well, presents with tingling and pain in her feet associated with abdominal pain and difficulty swallowing.

On examination she has a left facial weakness, both legs are weak and ataxic with reduced reflexes and downward plantars. Her upper limbs are normal.

Questions

(1) What investigations would you do?
(2) What is the most likely diagnosis?
(3) What is the likely outcome?

Question 97

A previously well 3-year-old is brought to casualty because she keeps falling over.

On examination she is ataxic and has difficulty talking.

Physical examination is normal. There is no family history of inherited neurological disease but her 10-year-old brother (from her father's previous marriage) does have convulsions.

Investigations

Hb	11.2 g/dl
WBC	$9.5 \times 10^9/l$
Platelets	$305 \times 10^9/l$
Sodium	135 mmol/l
Potassium	3.7 mmol/l
Calcium	2.1 mmol/l
Urea	4.2 mmol/l
Chloride	105 mmol/l
Bicarbonate	20 mmol/l
Glucose	6.3 mmol/l
Skull X-ray	normal

Questions

(1) What is the likely diagnosis?
(2) How would you confirm this?

Question 98

A 14-year-old boy presents in casualty with a persisting nose bleed. Over the last two weeks he has felt generally unwell with a sore throat and headache.

A week before he developed a rash that is now fading.
Investigation showed:

Hb	10.1 g/dl
Reticulocytes	4.8%
WBC	$19.7 \times 10^9/l$
neutrophils	45%
lymphocytes	35%
monocytes	18%
eosinophils	2%

Clotting	Patient	Control
PT(s)	15	14
PTT(K)(s)	41	38
Thrombin(s)	9	10
Fibrin	1/64	1/64

Questions

(1) What is the likely diagnosis?
(2) How would you confirm this?
(3) What further test would be useful?
(4) What further question would you like to ask?

Question 99

A 6-year-old girl is admitted following a generalized convulsion. Over the last 4 days she had complained of headache, and had become increasingly irritable and ataxic.

During several previous illnesses she had been drowsy, but eventually fully recovered. A male sibling had died at 2 weeks of age from an undiagnosed encephalopathy.

Investigations

Sodium	138 mmol/l
Potassium	4.2 mmol/l
Urea	3.8 mmol/l
Glucose	3.5 mmol/l

Serum bilirubin 9 μmol/l
AST 400 IU/l
ALT 850 IU/l
Serum ammonia 200 μmol/l (0–40 μmol/l)
Urine orotic acid/creatinine ratio: increased
CSF
  clear and colourless
  WBC 4×10^6/l
  protein 0.4 g/dl
  glucose 2.8 mmol/l

Questions

(1) What is the most likely diagnosis?
(2) Is there any connection with the death of the sibling?

Question 100

A healthy 10-year-old boy is noted to have a tachycardia after being given pre-medication for a routine surgical procedure.

Question

What abnormality is shown on the ECG?

Question 101

The following investigations are from a 16-year-old girl with aortic coarctation:

Height 120 cm
Weight 28 kg
LH (basal level) 40 IU/l
FSH (basal level) 30 IU/l
Plasma oestradiol <10 pmol/l
Bone age 11 years, osteoporosis noted on X-ray

Questions

(1) What is the probable diagnosis?
(2) What one investigation would confirm this?

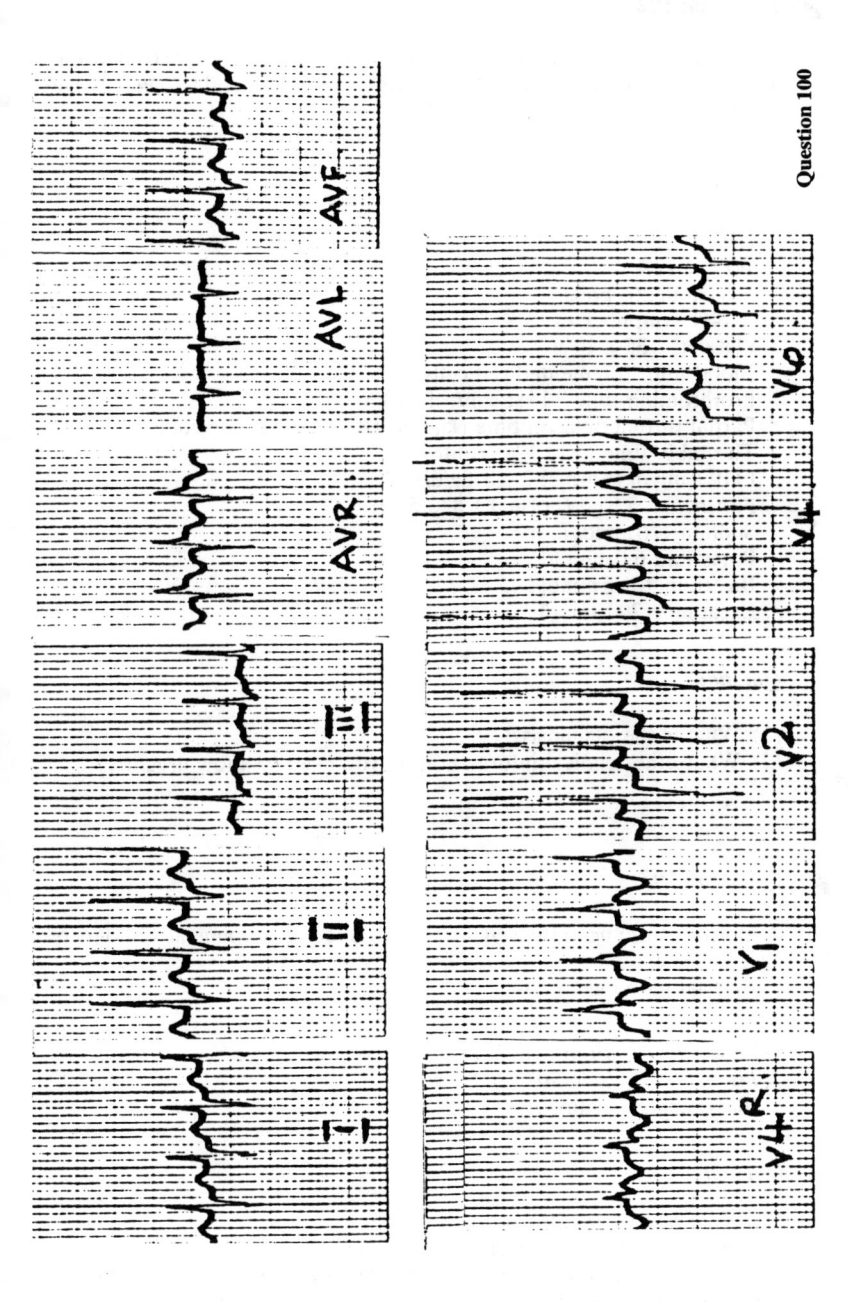

Question 100

Question 102

A 2-year-old boy is admitted to hospital following a grand mal convulsion. He has been listless and irritable for the last few days and a week ago had diarrhoea and vomiting lasting 4 days.

Investigations

HB 6.1 g/dl
WBC 12.1×10^9/l
  80% neutrophils
  14% lymphocytes
Platelets 35×10^9/l
Blood film: fragmented red cells
Prothrombin time 14 s; control 13.5 s
Partial thromboplastin time (kaolin) (PTTK) 45 s; control 38 s
Thrombin time (TT) 12 s; control 9 s
FDP 8 mg/dl (normal 2–10 mg/dl)
Fibrinogen 3.3 g/l (normal 1.8–3.5 g/l)
Sodium 126 mmol/l
Potassium 6.0 mmol/l
Bicarbonate 15 mmol/l
Creatinine 200 µmol/l

Questions

(1) What is the diagnosis?
(2) What other clinical information do you need to know urgently?

Question 103

A 'normal' term neonate weighing 3.4 kg is found 'gasping' at 12 hours of age.
  Arterial blood gas shows:

pH   7.04
P_{CO_2} 19 mmHg (2.5 kPa)
P_{O_2} 51 mmHg (6.8 kPa)
Bicarbonate 6 mmol/l

Questions

(1) What physiological abnormality is shown?
(2) What further clinical test should be performed?
(3) What important diagnosis should be considered in this situation?
(4) Name two other conditions that could present like this.

Question 104

A maladjusted boy of 8 years from a large family is noted to have progressively reduced visual acuity in his right eye on routine school screening.

He suffers from enuresis and recurrent bouts of bronchitis. His height is on the 50th centile and weight on the 25th centile.

On examination his liver is 3 cm below the right costal margin, and there is a white lesion over the macular area of his fundus on the right side.

Investigations

Hb	11 g/dl
WBC	$10 \times 10^9/l$
neutrophils	68%
lymphocytes	10%
monocytes	7%
eosinophils	15%

Questions

(1) What is the most likely diagnosis?
(2) Name three investigations.
(3) What advice would you give his parents?

Question 105

A male infant presents at 4 months of age weighing 3.8 kg. He had been a full-term normal delivery weighing 3.5 kg, was breast fed and always seemed to feed well.

On examination he was pale, oedematous and underweight, his chest X-ray showed patchy areas in the left upper lobe and the right middle lobe. Investigation showed:

Hb	7.1 g/dl
WBC	$19.0 \times 10^9/l$
Reticulocytes	4.5%
Bilirubin	97 μmol/l
Albumin	20 g/l

Questions

(1) Why is he anaemic?
(2) What is the underlying condition?
(3) What further single test would be diagnostic?

Question 106

A 14-month-old infant is investigated following an early morning convulsion.

    Random blood glucose 1.8 mmol/l
    Serum lipids
        triglyceride 3.5 mmol/l   0.6 — 1.7
        cholesterol 9.7 mmol/l   3.1 — 6.8

Question

What is the diagnosis?

Question 107

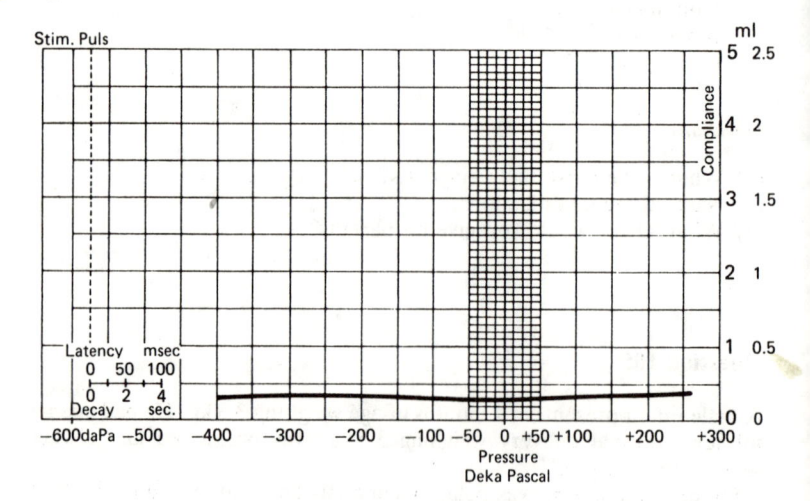

Questions

(1) What does this tympanogram demonstrate?
(2) What two conditions would give such a recording?
(3) What information is normally given that would differentiate these two conditions?

Question 108

A 4-year-old boy presents with a history of increasing diarrhoea over a 3-month period.

Today his mother noted he had 'puffy' eyes on waking: this was confirmed on examination and there was a suggestion of oedema around his ankles.

Initial investigation revealed:

Hb	11.1 g/dl
WBC	6.7×10^9/l
neutrophils	78%
lymphocytes	19%
monocytes	2%
Serum albumin	21 g/dl
Urine protein	30 mg/24 hours

Questions

(1) What is the likely diagnosis?
(2) How would you confirm this?

Question 109

A 9-year-old boy fell from a tree and received a chest injury. He was seen in casualty where a rib fracture was confirmed and he went home with analgesics.

Two months later he was referred by his GP because of increasing tiredness and exertional dyspnoea.

On examination he was noted to be tachycardic and slightly cyanosed. Cardiovascular and respiratory systems were otherwise normal.

Chest X-ray showed a lobular shadow in the right lower zone.

Investigations showed:

Hb	17.8 g/dl
PCV	64%
TLC	1600 ml
VC	1450 ml
Peak flow	260 l/min

Diffusion capacity: normal
Helium dilution time: normal

pH	7.43
Pco_2	38 mmHg (5.0 kPa)
Po_2	48 mmHg (6.4 kPa); post-100% O_2 saturation = 98%
Bicarbonate	21 mmol/l

Questions

(1) What is the physiological abnormality?
(2) What is the cause of this in this child?
(3) How would you confirm this?

Question 110

The following catheter data are from a 5-year-old boy with known cardiomyopathy.

	Oxygen saturation (%)	Pressure (mmHg)
Superior vena cava	44	
Right atrium	45	mean 16
Inferior vena cava	46	
Right ventricle	46	60/16
Pulmonary artery	45	60/39, mean 51
Pulmonary vein	92	
Left atrium	92	mean 20 (V-wave 30)
Left ventricle	92	90/22
Aorta	92	90/70, mean 80

Questions

(1) What abnormalities are present?
(2) What can you conclude from this study?

Question 111

A 7-year-old boy is investigated for precocious puberty and loss of conjugate eye movements.

Height 140 cm (>90th centile)
Testicular volume 18 ml
Bone age 12 years
LHRH stimulation test

	0 min	30 min	60 min
LH (IU/l)	6.0	11.0	15.0
FSH (IU/l)	1.0	1.8	2.4

Questions

(1) What is the most likely diagnosis?
(2) What further investigations are indicated?

Question 112

The following arterial blood gas results are from an 11-year-old girl with post-infective polyneuritis.

pH   7.26
P_{O_2} 9.2 kPa (69 mmHg)
P_{CO_2} 9.5 kPa (71 mmHg)

Questions

(1) What do these results show?
(2) What is the cause?
(3) What immediate treatment is required?

Question 113

A Turkish child on holiday in Britain presents with a cold, cough and wheeze.
  A full blood count reveals the following:

Hb   11.2 g/dl
WBC 5×10^9/l normal differential count
PCV   37%
RBC 5.3×10^9/l
MCV   67 fl
MCH   23.4 pg
MCHC   33.7 g/dl

The report reads: 'red cells are hypochromic and microcytic with poikilocytosis and some ovalocytes present'.

Questions

(1) What is the most likely diagnosis?
(2) What two further tests would you like to perform?

Question 114

A 5-year-old girl with ataxia has recurrent chest infections.
  Investigations were as follows:

Hb   12.4 g/dl
WBC 5.6×10^9/l
  55% neutrophils
  45% lymphocytes

Serum immunoglobulins (normal range for age in brackets):

IgG 100 IU/ml (63–160)
IgM 180 IU/ml (50–220)
IgA   2 IU/ml (25–117)
IgE   0 IU/ml (5–621)

Questions

(1) What is the diagnosis?
(2) What further physical signs might you expect to find?
(3) What further investigation might be helpful?

Question 115

A 12-year-old boy with a 3-day history of sore throat, headache and fever was treated by his general practitioner with co-trimoxazole. After an initial improvement he developed frequent episodes of vomiting and was admitted to hospital.

Investigations

Hb   13.5 g/dl
WBC $10.1 \times 10^9/l$
Platelets $240 \times 10^9/l$
Blood glucose   3.8 mmol/l
Chest X-ray   normal

Antibiotics were discontinued but over the following 24 hours he became disorientated and drowsy. A lumbar puncture at this time gave the following results:

CSF clear and colourless
  protein   0.8 g/dl
  glucose   2.6 mmol/l
  cells
    RBC $10 \times 10^6/l$
    WBC $380 \times 10^6/l$
      40% polymorphs
      60% lymphocytes
  Gram stain, no organisms seen

Questions

(1) What is the likely diagnosis?
(2) List three further investigations.

Question 116

An 8-year-old boy known to have a cystic fibrosis presents with increasing fatigue and breathlessness.
Results show:

Hb 13.1 g/dl
WBC $9.7 \times 10^9/l$
pH 7.31
P_{CO_2} 44 mmHg (5.8 kPa)
P_{O_2} 51 mmHg (6.8 kPa)
ECG reported as showing peaked Ps in II, III and aVF, and right ventricular hypertrophy

Questions

(1) Name two complications that can be inferred from these results.
(2) What is the first line in management?

Question 117

A bottle-fed 4-day-old term neonate is becoming increasingly jaundiced. The mother's previous child needed phototherapy and as a result the mother's blood type is already known.
The results are as follows:

Mother group O positive (CDe/CDe)
Baby group A positive
direct Coombs' positive
bilirubin 280 µmol/l

Questions

(1) Name two causes from the data presented.
(2) Can this be serious?
(3) How would you manage this infant?

Question 118

Questions

(1) Describe this EEG (*opposite*).
(2) What did the EEG staff notice about the patient during this recording?
(3) How might this patient have induced this ECG?

Question 118

Question 119

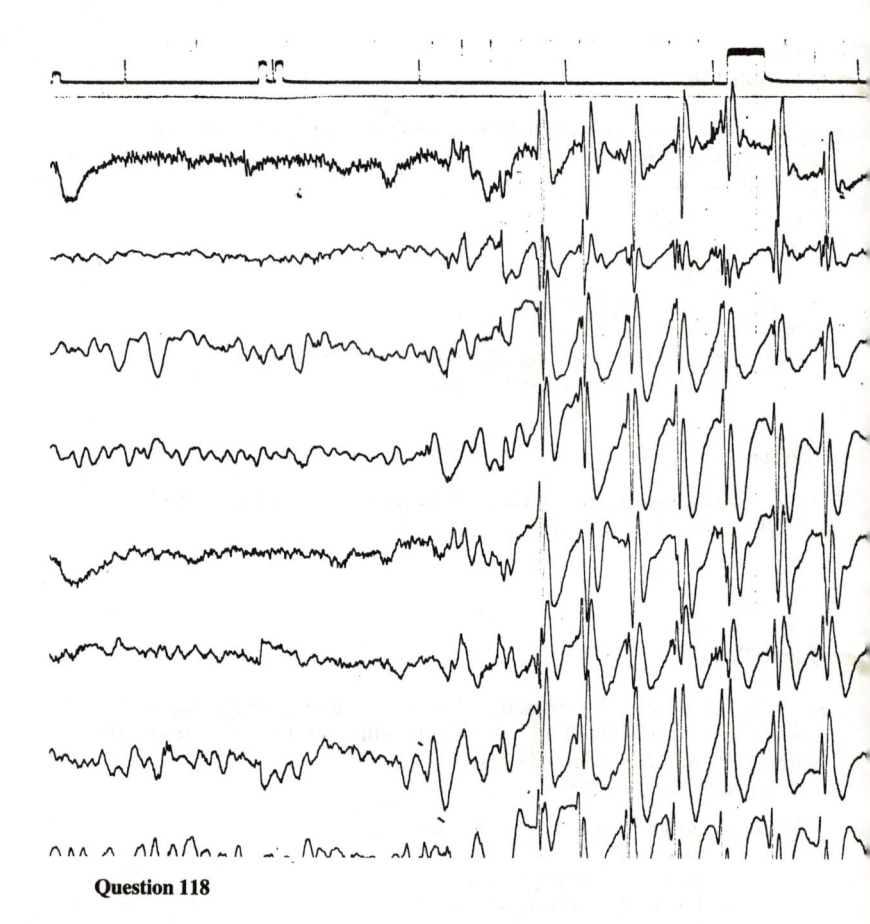

Three days after a normal spontaneous vaginal delivery at term, a 3.4-kg neonate has an apnoeic episode.
Investigation shows:

Sodium	140 mmol/l
Potassium	3.7 mmol/l
Creatinine	55 µmol/l
Calcium	2.0 mmol/l
Glucose	1.6 mmol/l
Clotting studies	normal

Questions

(1) What is the likely aetiology of the apnoeic episode?
(2) What further investigations would you perform?
(3) How would you manage this infant?

Question 120

Questions

(1) List three abnormalities shown on this ECG (*opposite*).
(2) What is the likely diagnosis?

Question 121

A 6-year-old boy is found to be hypertensive following admission to hospital for tonsillectomy.
On examination

Height 30th centile
Weight >97th centile
BP   160/95
Facial acne and hypertrichosis present

Investigations

Hb 17.8 g/dl
Skull X-ray normal
Bone age 7 years
Urinary 17-ketosteroids 40 μmol/24 h (normal 0–8.7)
Urinary 17-hydroxycorticosteroids 42 μmol/24 h (normal 21–28)
Midnight cortisol 85% of 09:00 level
High dose dexamethasone suppression test (2 mg 6-hourly):
  no suppression

Questions

(1) What is the probable diagnosis?
(2) What two investigations would you do next?
(3) What is the treatment?

Question 122

A premature baby born at 30 weeks' gestation is seen routinely at term in the outpatient department with the following routine tests having been performed. The child is asymptomatic.

Weight   2.6 kg
Hb   12.3 g/dl
WBC 10.7×10^9/l
RBC 3.2×10^{12}/l
MCH   32 pg
Sodium   137 mmol/l

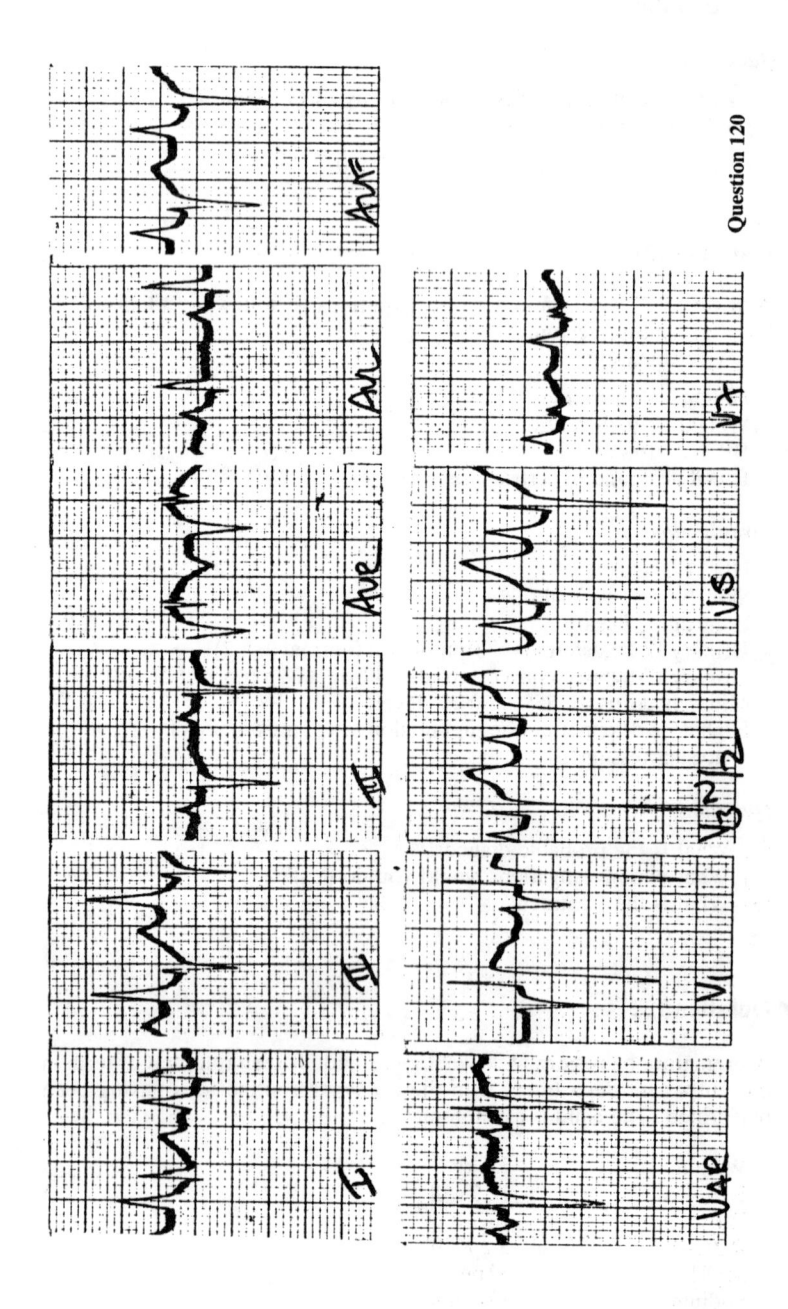

Question 120

Potassium	4.2 mmol/l
Chloride	91 mmol/l
Calcium	2.14 mmol/l =
Phosphate	1.15 mmol/l =
Alkaline phosphatase	2042 IU/l ↑
Magnesium	0.9 mmol/l =

Questions

(1) What is the diagnosis?
(2) Are there any further tests required?
(3) What is the management?

Question 123

The following investigations, including the EEG on p. 68, are from a 10-year-old boy.

Hb	10.2 g/dl
WBC	3.0×10^9/l
RBC	3.2×10^{12}/l
MCV	104 fl
MCH	32 pg
MCHC	31 g/dl
Platelets	100×10^9/l

Questions

(1) What are the two major abnormalities shown?
(2) What is the likely connection between these?

Question 124

A 3-year-old boy is admitted to hospital with a chest infection. He has always been a difficult feeder and his weight is on the 3rd centile. He is clumsy and his language development is delayed.

On examination he is noted to have cold hands (despite reasonable blood pressure), acrocyanosis, and is sweating. His knee and ankle reflexes are absent.

The chest X-ray as well as showing some pneumonic changes also shows a rib fracture.

Questions

(1) What is the diagnosis?
(2) What tests confirm the diagnosis?
(3) What is the prognosis?

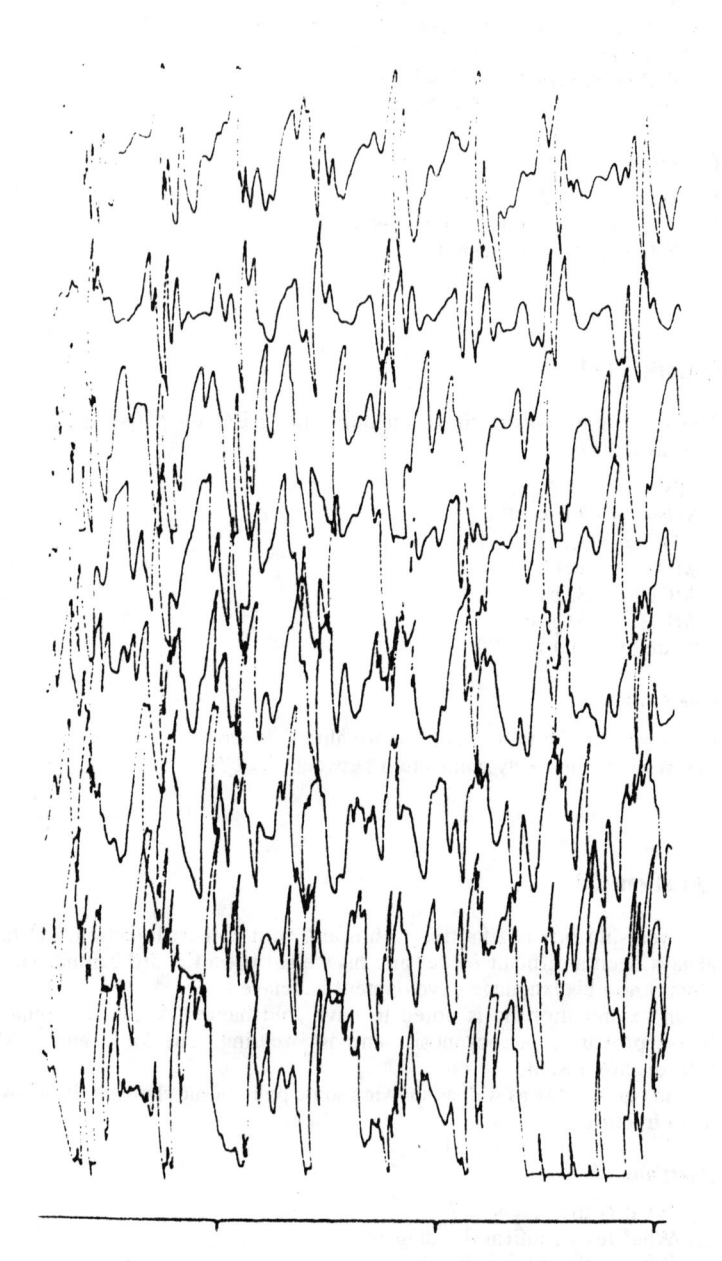

Question 123

Question 125

A 15-year-old haemophiliac presents with abdominal pain and painful movement of his right hip.

Questions

(1) What is the diagnosis?
(2) How would you confirm this?
(3) What levels of factor VIII are needed to manage this problem?

Question 126

A 12-year-old boy is admitted to hospital systemically unwell with a fever, tachypnoea and intermittent cough.
His full blood count shows:

Hb	8.3 g/dl ↓
PCV	31%
MCHC	34 g/dl
MCV	88 fl (μm^3)
RBC	3 × 10^{12}/l ↓
WBC	48 × 10^9/l ↑↑
neutrophils	65%
metamyelocytes	12%
myelocytes	6%
basophils	1%
eosinophils	1%
lymphocytes	15%
Platelets	160 × 10^9/l

The film shows polychromasia with anisocytes and poikilocytes present.

Questions

(1) Describe this blood picture.
(2) What is the most likely cause in this child?
(3) Name three other causes.

Question 127

A child draws the following 'Mummy' and 'house'.

Question

How old would you expect this child to be?

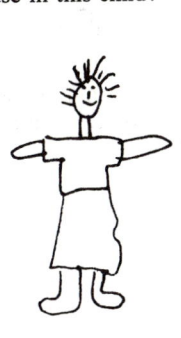

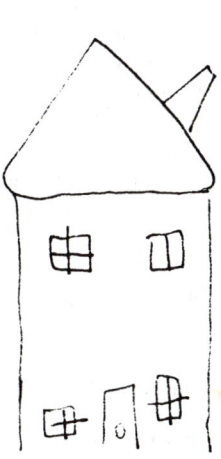

Question 128

A 9-year-old is referred with brown cloudy urine. The child is otherwise well and says this has happened three or four times before but he has never told anyone.

On examination he appears healthy and his blood pressure is normal. Investigations show:

Urine
    RBC   400 per high power field
    WBC   25 per high power field
    no casts
    protein   1+
    culture   no growth
Plasma
    sodium   138 mmol/l
    potassium   4.1 mmol/l
    urea   3.7 mmol/l
Haematology
    Hb   14.1 g/dl
    WBC 11.2×10^9/l
    platelets 360×10^9/l
    ESR   3 mm/h
    Complement 0.9 g/dl (normal range 0.89–2.09 g/dl)

Questions

(1) Name two diagnoses.
(2) What further history would be useful?
(3) Give two further investigations that may be useful.

Question 129

A 5-year-old girl is investigated for hypertension.

On examination her blood pressure is 145/95 and she has ambiguous genitalia.

The following abnormal results were obtained:

Serum sodium   150 mmol/l
Urinary pregnanetriol   6 µmol/24 h (normal <3.3)
Serum 11-deoxycortisol 900 ng/dl (normal levels 200–500 ng/dl)

Question

What is the diagnosis?

Question 130

The ECG indicated is from a 10-month-old girl with Down's syndrome.

Question 130

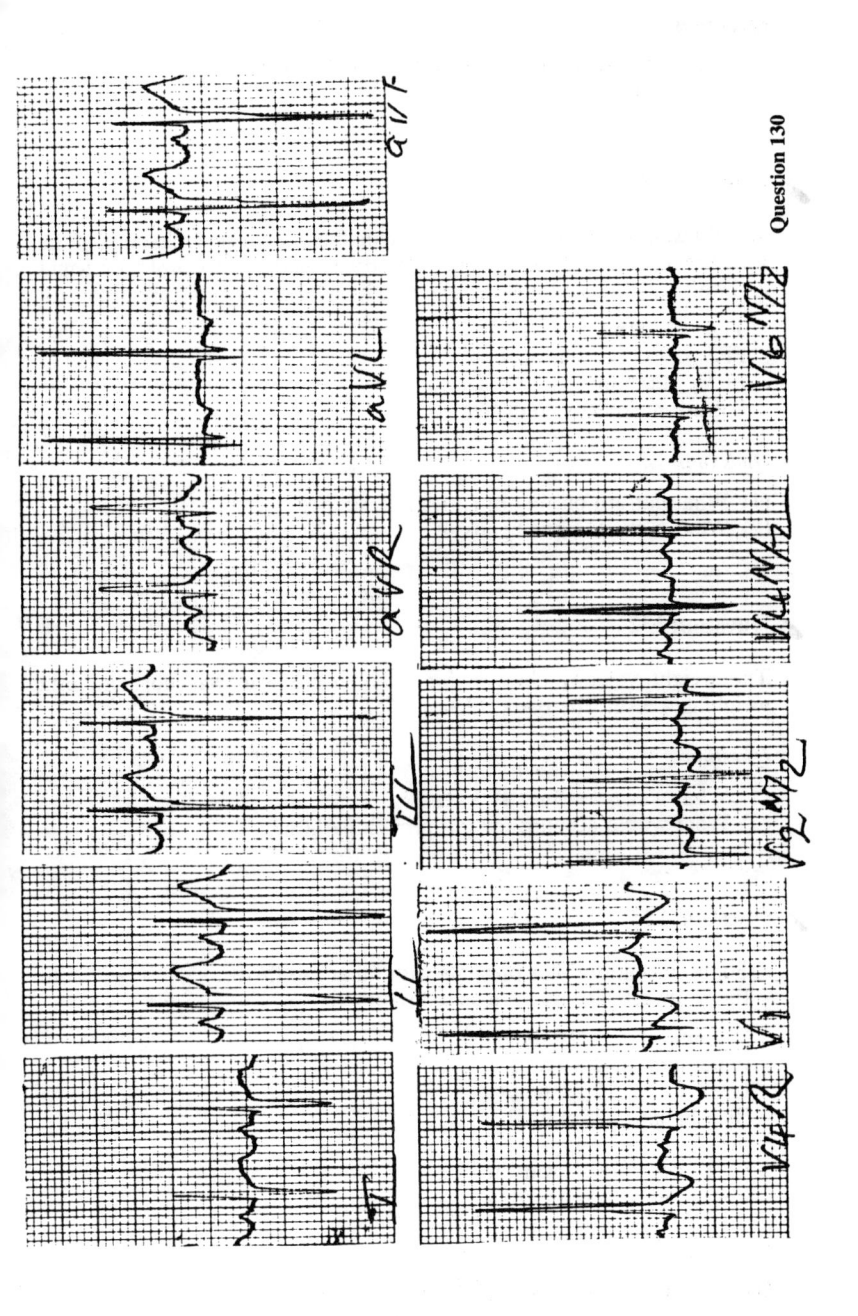

Questions

(1) What abnormalities are present on this ECG?
(2) What is the diagnosis?

Question 131

A child was successfully treated for acute lymphoblastic leukaemia at the age of two and a half. At the age of 18 he was on the 50th centile for height and weight, at which time the following lung function tests were obtained:

↓ TLC   2500 ml
   FEV_1/FVC ratio normal
↓ FEV_1 2000 ml
   Diffusion capacity: reduced

Questions

(1) What pattern of abnormalities is described?
(2) What is the likely diagnosis?

Question 132

The weight velocity chart is for a 7-year-old who was born at term weighing 4.5 kg. The cord pH was 7.05.

Questions

(1) What was his weight at 3 years?
(2) What would account for this growth pattern?

Question 133

A 30-month-old toddler presents with failure to thrive.
Initial investigations were as follows:

Sodium   129 mmol/l
Potassium   2.3 mmol/l
Urea   2.7 mmol/l
Bicarbonate   35 mmol/l
pH   7.45
Urine negative on ward testing
His blood pressure is 70/40

Questions

(1) What is the diagnosis?
(2) Suggest three lines of management.

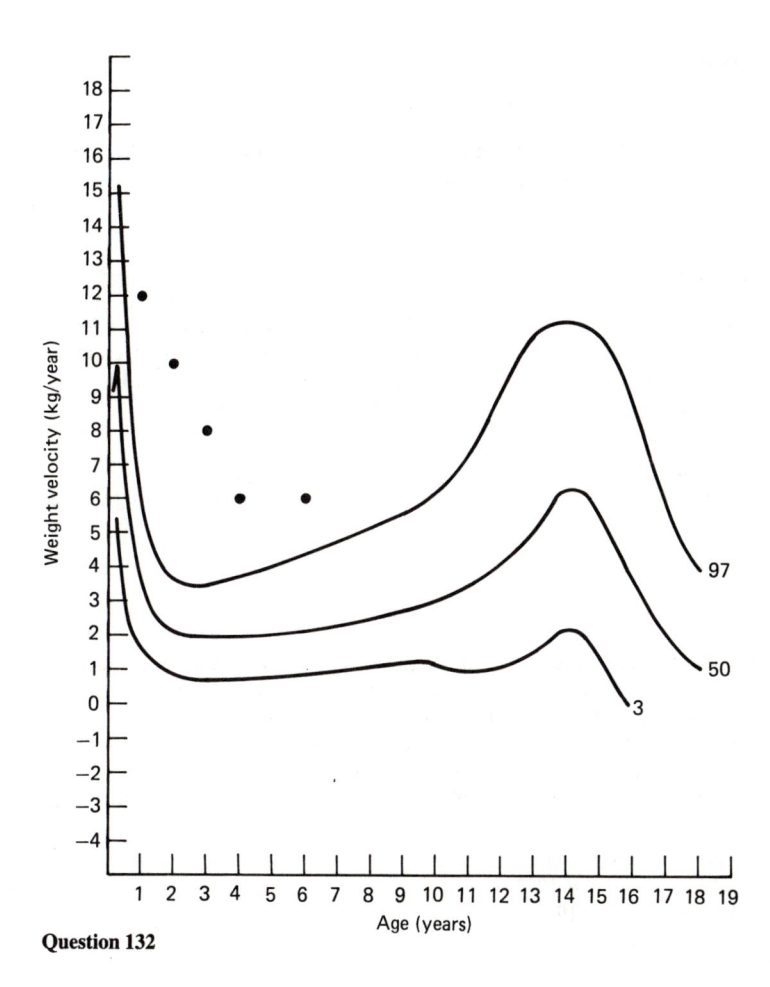

Question 132

Question 134
An obese 14-year-old presents with increasing lethargy. On examination she seems drowsy, is slightly cyanosed and her weight is well above the 97th centile.

Lung function tests show:

FEV$_1$ 1.4 l
Vital capacity 1.6 l
Total lung capacity 2.3 l
Diffusion capacity normal
Arterial blood gases:
  pH 7.34
  P_{CO_2} 65 mmHg (8.7 kPa)
  P_{O_2} 50 mmHg (6.7 kPa)

Questions

(1) What physiological abnormality is present?
(2) What biochemical abnormality is present?
(3) What is the probable cause of this child's abnormalities?
(4) How would you manage this problem?

Question 135

The second child of normal healthy parents is discovered to have a meningomyelocele associated with hydrocephalus. Their first child had had a meningocele successfully repaired in the newborn period.

Questions

(1) What is the recurrence risk for the next sibling?
(2) What advice would you give these parents about future pregnancies?

Question 136

A full-term male infant, birth weight 4.7 kg, was delivered by emergency lower segment caesarean section because of fetal distress. Apart from being irritable, his first day examination was normal.
On day 7 he fed poorly and vomited twice. His urine output was poor and the urine was noted to be blood stained.
Examination revealed an unwell baby with a mass in the right flank.
Initial investigations:

Hb   16.5 g/dl
WBC $19.3 \times 10^9/l$
Platelets $33 \times 10^9/l$
Urine red cells +++

Questions

(1) What is the most likely diagnosis?
(2) Give two other possible causes
(3) What further tests would you perform?
(4) Are any tests indicated for his mother?

Question 137

An 8-month-old infant who is irritable and feeding poorly presents because of a swelling on the left side of his face.
On examination the swelling is maximal over the mandible. The rectal temperature is 38.9°C and there is limited movement of the right arm.

Investigation shows:

Hb	8.4 g/dl normocytic film
WBC	24.6 × 10⁹/l
80% polymorphs	
Platelets	480 × 10⁹/l
ESR	42 mm/h
Urine protein	0.3 g/l

Questions

(1) What is the most likely diagnosis?
(2) What other diagnosis should be considered?
(3) Name two investigations.

Question 138

Intracerebral calcification is seen on the skull X-ray of a 3-year-old performed as a routine following a head injury after the child fell from a climbing frame.
The child's general health and development appears to be normal.

Questions

(1) What is the most likely cause?
(2) What further investigation is indicated?

Question 139

The following cardiac catheter data are from a 16-year-old girl.

	Oxygen saturation (%)	Pressure (mmHg)
Superior vena cava	65	
Right atrium	68	mean 11
Inferior vena cava	69	
Right ventricle	68	90/0–11
Pulmonary artery	67	90/60 mean 77
Pulmonary vein	100	
Left atrium	98	mean 10
Left ventricle	82	90/0–11
Aorta	78	90/62 mean 79

Questions

(1) What is the diagnosis?
(2) Is surgical correction required?

Answers and Discussion

Answer 1

(1) Shortened P–R interval.
    Delta wave.
    Widened QRS complex.
(2) Wolff–Parkinson–White syndrome.

Discussion

Wolff–Parkinson–White (WPW) syndrome results from an anomalous connection between atria and ventricles. This connection bypasses the AV node, hence the shortened P–R interval. There is early but slower depolarization of the ventricle to which it is connected (pre-excitation) and this causes the initial slurring of the QRS complex – the delta wave. The remainder of the ventricular system is depolarized in the normal way via the Purkinje system, but the net result is a widened QRS complex. Since ventricular depolarization is asynchronous, voltage criteria cannot be used to diagnose ventricular hypertrophy in the Wolff–Parkinson–White syndrome

In this ECG the P–R interval is 0.06 s (lower limit of normal for age, 0.10 s), the QRS duration is between 0.08 and 0.10 s (upper limit of normal for age, 0.06 s) with an obvious delta wave at the beginning of each complex. The heart rate is 115 beats/min and the rhythm is sinus. The QRS axis is approximately +30.

Children with Wolff–Parkinson–White syndrome may suffer from recurrent supraventricular tachyarrhythmias, most commonly re-entry tachycardias. In these, the accessory fibres allow retrograde conduction but, during the tachycardia, pre-excitation does not occur and hence the QRS complex is normal. Atrial fibrillation and flutter are both very rare in childhood Wolff–Parkinson–White syndrome, although a little more frequent in adolescents and adults.

In a minority of cases Wolff–Parkinson–White syndrome is associated with structural abnormalities, most commonly Ebstein's anomaly and mitral valve prolapse. The prognosis in children without structural defects is good and most respond to medical treatment. Surgical interruption of the accessory pathway is indicated if arrythmias are serious and resistant to medication.

Further reading

PARK, M. K. and GUNTHEROTH, W. G. (1981) *How to Read Pediatric ECGs*. Chicago: Year Book Medical Publishers Inc.

Answer 2

(1) Buccal pigmentation and pigmentation of skin creases.
(2) Addison's disease – simultaneous ACTH and cortisol.
(3) Autoimmune.
(4) Infusion of normal saline and hydrocortisone.
(5) Steroid replacement therapy.

Discussion

The pigmentation in Addison's disease, unlike suntanning, also affects hands, axillae, skin creases and nipples. The blood pressure should also be recorded – it is likely to be low.

Biochemical pointers toward this diagnosis are: low sodium, slightly raised potassium (check not haemolysed) and a low blood sugar. The raised urea reflects hypovolaemia. The urine osmolality divided by the calculated serum osmolality, i.e. $2 \times (Na^+ + K^+) + glucose + urea$, is greater than 1.1, thus excluding renal failure.

The ideal test is to measure ACTH and cortisol simultaneously – the ACTH will be high (diurnal rhythm will have been abolished) and cortisol low.

It should be noted that Addison's disease in childhood is very rare. The vague and non-specific symptoms of which this patient complained are not uncommon, however, and will more usually be found to be due to low grade infection of some kind.

The majority (50%) appear to be autoimmune in origin. This may be associated with multiple endocrinopathy associated with candidiasis (MEDAC) syndrome which also includes alopecia, hypoparathyroidism and pancreatic insufficiency.

Another group is HLA-B8 associated and shows a propensity toward autoimmune thyroid disease and insulin-dependent diabetes.

Tuberculosis is no longer the commonest cause but it should be excluded.

The underlying problem is not fully understood; defective suppressor T-cell function has been noted in some patients.

Initial management consists of a resuscitative dose of normal saline (10–20 ml/kg) plus dextrose if hypoglycaemic.

Blood for investigation should be taken before administration of hydrocortisone.

Long-term replacement therapy can be either cortisone acetate (four times daily) or prednisone (twice daily). These must be increased at times of stress.

Growth, ACTH, blood pressure and potassium should be monitored on a regular basis.

Monitoring of other endocrine gland function (especially thyroid) is advisable, together with checking other family members.

Further reading

BROOK, C. D. (Ed.) (1981) *Clinical Paediatric Endocrinology* p. 410. Oxford: Blackwell Scientific
FORFAR, P. 1132
NELSON, p. 1478

Answer 3

(1) Bodian–Shwachman syndrome.
(2) Pancreatic function tests; sweat test.
(3) Pancreatic replacement therapy and antibiotics for intercurrent infection.

Discussion

Bodian–Shwachman syndrome – the history suggests failure to thrive secondary to a gastrointestinal disorder. Investigation reveals a neutropenia (which is a repeatable finding) and there are minor hepatic enzyme changes. These findings, together with the absence of respiratory problems, suggest the second commonest cause of exocrine pancreatic deficiency after cystic fibrosis. Nevertheless the incidence is only about 1 or 2 per 200 000.

The underlying disorder has been postulated to be a cellular microtubular or microfilament problem leading to widespread tissue involvement. The full syndrome may include: growth retardation; bone marrow hypoplasia – neutropenia, thrombocytopenia; raised HbF; a tendency toward lymphoproliferative neoplasia; skeletal dysostoses; hepatomegaly and renal tubular dysfunction.

Further reading

AGGETT, P. J. et al., (1980) Shwachman syndrome. Archives of the Diseases of Childhood, **55**, 331
NELSON, P. 1240
SHWACHMAN, H., DYAMOND, I. K., OSKI, F. A. and KON'T KHAW (1964) The syndrome of pancreatic insufficiency and bone marrow dysfunction. *Journal of pediatrics*, **65**, 645

Answer 4

(1) Hypocalcaemic tetany.
(2) Alkaline phosphatase; X-ray wrist.
(3) Intravenous calcium gluconate.

Discussion

Sudden onset of stridor may be due to inhalation of a foreign body; however, the serum calcium is low and phosphorus very low – suggesting prolonged deficiency of vitamin D. In the early stages of rickets, calcium is low and phosphorus maintained.

Toddler rickets may occur due to displacement from the breast by the next sibling and an ensuing poor intake – the low haemoglobin also suggests this.

More commonly rickets presents with a bow-legged gait. The alkaline phosphatase is raised and the wrist X-ray shows flaring of the metaphysis – the classical radiological picture. A lateral X-ray of neck may be needed to exclude a foreign body.

Initial therapy should be intravenous 10% calcium gluconate (0.3 ml/kg, diluted to a 2–5% solution) slowly under cardiac monitoring conditions. This can be followed by either one very large dose of vitamin D, e.g. 6 000 000 U, or this dose divided over the following weeks combined with education of the parents to provide a balanced diet.

Further reading

FORFAR, P. 1299
NELSON, P. 249

Answer 5

(1) Lactic acidosis.
(2) Assay blood lactate.

Discussion

The obvious abnormality in these electrolytes is the very low bicarbonate, which, with this history, is almost certainly attributable to a severe metabolic acidosis. The second abnormality is the large 'anion gap'. Blood has no net electrical charge; the sum of the cations must equal that of the anions. Sodium ions constitute essentially almost all of the cations while chloride, bicarbonate, phosphate, sulphate, proteins and organic acids make up the majority of the anions. Of these sodium, chloride and bicarbonate are the only ions routinely measured; the 'anion gap' is the difference between these, i.e. $Na^+ - [Cl^- + HCO_3^-]$. Normally this is 12–15 mmol/l, but in the presence of excess unmeasured anions may be considerably higher. This boy has an anion gap of 38 mmol/l. The most likely cause of a metabolic acidosis with an increased anion gap in a child with septicaemic shock is an acquired lactic acidosis associated with ketoacidosis. Poor tissue perfusion leads to cellular hypoxia and a rise in lactate, due to both increased production, primarily from glycolysis, and decreased utilization. Lactic acidosis is also associated with inborn errors of gluconeogenesis and of pyruvate oxidation (e.g. glucose-6-phosphatase deficiency and pyruvate carboxylase deficiency). Congenital organic acidaemias (e.g. propionic acidaemia) cause accumulation of other organic acids but can be associated with lactic acidosis. An increased anion gap may also be caused by exogenous compounds such as salicylates, paraldehyde, methanol, and ethylene glycol.

Blood lactate levels should be less than 2 mmol/l, but levels up to 5 mmol/l may be normal (children who are upset and struggling may have increased blood levels). In this child, 3-hydroxybutyrate and acetocetate ('ketone bodies') will also be raised.

Further reading

COHEN, F. D. and WOODS, H. F. (1976) *Clinical Aspects of Lactic Acidosis.* Oxford: Blackwell Scientific Publications

Answer 6

(1) von Willebrand's disease.
(2) Assay factor VIIIWF, factor VIIIc and factor VIIIag. Platelet function (ristocetin aggregation).
(3) Inheritance is autosomal dominant.
(4) He should wear a 'medic alert' bracelet, and inform any dentists and doctors responsible for his care.

Discussion

von Willebrand's disease is a disorder characterized by abnormalities of factor VIII and platelet aggregation. Platelet numbers are normal and inheritance is autosomal dominant. The severity is variable, 25% of patients having purpura, but bleeding is most commonly from mucous membranes. Haemarthrosis is not characteristic.

Factor VIII is isolated from plasma as part of an aggregate of proteins of total molecular weight 20×10^6. Pure factor VIII has a molecular weight of 320 000. Factor VIIIc and factor VIIIcag are assays of the clotting activity and the antigenic properties, respectively. The aggregate also contains von Willebrand factor (VWF) of molecular weight 220 000 assayed as factor VIIIWF and VIIIRag (factor VIII related antigen).

Factor VIIIc is reduced in both von Willebrand's disease and haemophilia A and B. Factor VIIIcag, assayed by an immunoradioassay, is normal in haemophilia B (Christmas disease), but reduced in haemophilia A and von Willebrand's disease. Factor VIIIRag and factor VIIIWF are both high or normal in haemophilia but reduced in von Willebrand's disease. Factor VIIIWF is necessary for normal platelet function and, in von Willebrand's disease, platelet adhesion and platelet aggregation with ristocetin is abnormal. The bleeding time is normal in haemophilia.

Specific treatment for von Willebrand's disease is usually only required prior to surgery or dental extraction. When minor or major surgery is contemplated 2–4 bags of cryoprecipitate should be given every 12 hours for two days to restore haemostasis to normal. Fresh frozen plasma is effective but larger volumes are required for the same effect.

Further reading

BLOOM, A. L. and PEAKE, I. R. (1977) Factor VIII and its inherited disorders. *British Medical Bulletin*, **33**, 219–214
FORFAR, P. 969
NACHMAN, R. L. (1977) von Willebrand's disease and the molecular pathology of haemostasis. *New England Journal of Medicine*, 1059
NELSON, P. 1246

Answer 7

(1) Hereditary spherocytosis.
(2) Autohaemolysis test.

Discussion

To answer this question confidently, one needs to be aware that up to 20% of cases of hereditary spherocytosis are sporadic; there will not, therefore, always be the usual family history suggesting autosomal dominant inheritance.

Spherocytes are characteristic of both hereditary spherocytosis and autoimmune haemolytic anaemia. They are also seen in septicaemia caused by *Clostridium welchii* in burns patients and following blood transfusions. In this child the main differential diagnosis is between hereditary spherocytosis and autoimmune haemolytic anaemia. The latter is ruled out by a negative Coombs' test.

The cause of hereditary spherocytosis is thought to be an abnormality of the cytoskeleton of the red cell membrane. Sodium influx into the red cell is increased up to 50% above normal but this is not diagnostic in itself. The spherocyte is a more rigid structure than the normal red cell and is easily damaged as it passes through the spleen.

Hereditary spherocytosis can be confirmed by the autohaemolysis test in which blood is incubated at 37°C for 48 hours. Normal red cells show less than 5% haemolysis, in hereditary spherocytosis the figure is between 15% and 45%. The spherocytes fragment as glucose, required for the 'cation pump', is used up. If exogenous glucose is added prior to incubation this phenomenon is abolished. The osmotic fragility test is not specific for hereditary spherocytosis and is, therefore, not a satisfactory answer.

Patients may present with jaundice in the neonatal period when hereditary spherocytosis may be difficult to differentiate from ABO incompatibility. During childhood the anaemia is usually mild. The majority of children appear jaundiced. Complications include the development of pigmentary gallstones (but these do not usually develop until adolesence) and, more seriously, aplastic crises. Splenectomy cures the haemolytic anaemia, but in view of the known dangers of splenectomy this is best delayed until late childhood if possible.

Further reading

NELSON, PP. 1218–1219
WILEY, J. S. (1983) The haemolytic anaemias. *Medicine International*, **1**, 1202–1206

Chol 3-5.5
TGs 0.35-1

Answer 8

(1) Abetalipoproteinaemia
(2) Absence of β-lipoprotein on plasma electrophoresis.
(3) Low fat diet: medium chain triglycerides substituted for long chain triglycerides; fat-soluble vitamins with very high doses of vitamin E.

Discussion

Abetalipoproteinaemia is a rare disorder in which there is a defect in the production of apoprotein B by the cells of the intestine. This results in defective synthesis of low-density lipoproteins (LDL), very low-density lipoproteins (VLDL), and chylomicrons. Lipids cannot be transported from the intestine or liver. Inheritance is autosomal recessive. Absence of chylomicrons leads to malabsorption of fat and fat-soluble vitamins. The initial presentation is usually that of steatorrhoea. Cholesterol levels are very low, usually less than 1.3 mmol/l (normal range 3.0–5.5 mmol/l) with triglyceride levels less than 0.17 mmol/l (normal range 0.35–1.0 mmol/l). Acanthocytes are present from birth but are not diagnostic since they may also be found following splenectomy and in malabsorptive states. Vitamin K deficiency may lead to hypoprothrombinaemia. Children with this condition develop, after the first decade, a progressive ataxia and retinitis pigmentosa. Prolonged vitamin E deficiency appears to be primarily responsible for the neurological abnormalities. Diagnosis is strongly suggested by the combination of steatorrhoea, acanthocytosis and very low cholesterol and triglyceride levels. This is confirmed by the absence of β-lipoprotein on serum lipoprotein electrophoresis. On intestinal biopsy the epithelial cells show characteristic morphological changes, being swollen and fat laden. The villous architecture is normal, and there is no inflammatory infiltrate.

Treatment consists of a low fat diet with fat-soluble vitamins. Vitamin E, given in large enough doses to correct red cell peroxide haemolysis, is thought to prevent the development of neurological disease. Normal plasma vitamin A levels should be maintained and the prothrombin time corrected with sufficient vitamin K. Rickets does not usually occur as normal vitamin D intake appears adequate.

Further reading

LLOYD, J. K. (1984) Plasma lipid disorders. In *Chemical Pathology in the Sick Child*, edited by B. E. Clayton and J. M. Round, pp. 245–264. Oxford: Blackwell Scientific Publications

Answer 9

(1) Jaundice associated with breast feeding.
(2) Infection.
(3) Repeat bilirubin estimations.

Discussion

Jaundice in the newborn period does not necessarily infer a pathological process; indeed about 60% of term and 80% of preterm infants are noted to be jaundiced in the first week of life.

The decision to investigate a baby who is jaundiced therefore depends upon:

(1) The time of onset.
(2) The rate of rise of bilirubin.
(3) The 'type', i.e. conjugated or unconjugated.
(4) The actual value.
(5) The duration of jaundice.

Jaundice in the first 24 hours of life is generally considered pathological until proved otherwise – there is either increased breakdown of red cells, for example, haemolysis, or very rarely a problem of uptake (transient familial neonatal hyperbilirubinaemia).

The rate of rise is usually plotted on 'standard' charts (e.g. see Cockington, 1979) depending on the birth weight and gestation of the infant. The charts generally indicate when phototherapy and exchange transfusion should be considered in the well baby – these guidelines are reduced for an infant who is ill, shocked, hypothermic, hypoglycaemic or acidotic. Where the rate of rise is steeper than the 'accepted' line, then again haemolysis should be excluded.

Infection should always be considered as it is one process which is easily treated and failure to treat may be fatal.

Unconjugated hyperbilirubinaemia is associated with kernicterus – the bilirubin is fat soluble rather than water soluble, having not been conjugated prior to excretion. Conjugated bilirubin is generally a small proportion of the total bilirubin in the newborn because once conjugated it is promptly excreted. The management of conjugated hyperbilirubinaemia is discussed under 'biliary atresia'.

The significance of the actual value depends on the age of the child – levels of 200 μmol/l are significant on the first day, but not day 5 for a term infant – once again refer to the charts.

'Physiological' jaundice generally has disappeared by days 10–14. Investigation of prolonged jaundice may include TORCH screen, Australia antigen status, α_1-antitrypsin, serum and urine amino acids, a sweat test, and thyroid function tests.

This infant's investigations show no signs of haemolysis and no sign of liver dysfunction – note that haemoglobulin levels and the Coombs' test can be normal in ABO incompatibility.

As this child is 5 days old, and breast feeding well, the most likely diagnosis is jaundice associated with breast milk. It has been suggested that 5β-pregnane-3α,20β-diol and non-esterified long chain fatty acids inhibit glucuronyl transferase activity and so inhibit bilirubin uptake in the liver – resulting in jaundice. The jaundice rapidly subsides on discontinuing breast feeding for 24–48 hours.

Jaundice at this level in a well term infant at 5 days is not associated with long-term morbidity and is therefore not an indication for phototherapy. The role of phototherapy is to prevent the need for an exchange transfusion – it would not be expected that this child's jaundice would continue to rise to exchange levels.

Continued monitoring of serum bilirubin is indicated until the child is over the 'peak' – if levels do continue to rise then phototherapy would be indicated.

Further reading

COCKINGTON, R. A. (1979) A guide to the use of phototherapy in the management of neonatal hyperbilirubinaemia. *Journal of pediatrics*, **95**, 281–285
NELSON, pp. 356, 380

Answer 10

(1) Ventricular septal defect with left to right shunt.
    Moderate pulmonary arterial hypertension.
(2) Digoxin and diuretics if in heart failure.
    Antibiotic prophylaxis against bacterial endocarditis.
    Surgical closure of the ventricular septal defect.

Discussion

There is a significant step-up in oxygen saturation between the right atrium and right ventricle, indicating shunting at ventricular level. Right ventricular and pulmonary artery pressures are significantly raised and therefore this is likely to be a ventricular septal defect (VSD) with a large left to right shunt. The ratio of pulmonary blood flow (Qp) to systemic blood flow (Qs) can be calculated using the following formula:

Qp = systemic arterial O_2 content − mixed systemic venous O_2 content
Qs = pulmonary venous O_2 content − pulmonary arterial O_2 content

So in this case the Qp/Qs ratio is approximately 3:1.

The majority of ventricular septal defects are small, asymptomatic and either close or decrease in size spontaneously. With large defects the degree and direction of shunting is dependent on the pulmonary vascular resistance (unless pulmonary stenosis is also present). Moderate and large shunts may cause heart failure which can often be successfully treated with medication. Bacterial endocarditis is not an uncommon complication and antibiotic prophylaxis is therefore important for dental or other procedures than can lead to infective endocarditis. Surgery is reserved for those who either:

(1) Fail to respond to medical treatment.
(2) Have a pulmonary to systemic flow (Qp/Qs) of >2:1.
(3) Have a Qp/Qs of <2:1, but have pulmonary hypertension.

(4) Have right ventricular pressure at systemic levels because of right ventricular outflow obstruction.

Surgery is contraindicated if Eisenmenger's syndrome (i.e. irreversible pulmonary vascular disease) has developed.

Further reading

JORDAN, S. C. and SCOTT, O. (1981) *Heart Disease in Paediatrics*, pp. 75–91. London: Butterworths

OAKLEY, C. (1980) Ventricular septal defects. In *Heart Disease in Infants and Children*, edited by G. Graham and E. Rossi, pp. 209–231. London: Edward Arnold

Answer 11

(1) About 240 mosmol/kg.
(2) Inappropriate antidiuretic hormone syndrome (SIADH).
(3) Urinary electrolytes and osmolality.
(4) Restrict fluids – include sodium in fluids.

Discussion

Inappropriate secretion of antidiuretic hormone (ADH) most commonly follows intracerebral pathology (meningitis, encephalitis or surgery etc.); however, it can follow any serious infection or surgical procedure, and following certain drugs, e.g. vincristine. Certain malignant tumours, e.g. Ewing's sarcoma, can produce ectopic ADH.

Water intoxication is the main differential diagnosis in this situation; always review the fluid balance charts yourself – what the child should get and does get can be quite dissimilar! Presuming this child has received the stated fluids then water intoxication is not likely, although the serum sodium might be low. In this situation one would expect the urine to be maximally dilute with little sodium loss; however, in inappropriate antidiuretic hormone syndrome this is not true and the finding of urine which has a relatively high osmolarity is diagnostic.

Management is primarily to restrict fluids; hypertonic saline (1.5%) is only indicated when the child is comatose or convulsing.

The role of demeclocycline is not established in childhood.

The calculated sum of the molar concentrations of the osmotically active particles in the plasma ($2 \times [Na^+ + K^+]$ + glucose + urea) is approximately equal to the plasma osmolality. It is only an approximation for two reasons. First, because of the high concentrations of sodium and chloride occurring in the plasma, some particles will be associated and so act as a single osmotically active particle. Secondly, protein particles occupy some of the volume contained in one litre of fluid, i.e. it is not pure solute.

In practice the major anions and cations make up 93% of plasma osmolality.

Further reading

FORFAR, pp. 400, 1110
NELSON, pp. 245, 630, 1440

Answer 12

(1) Renovascular hypertension with secondary hyperaldosteronism.
(2) Right renal artery stenosis (RAS) or branch stenosis.
(3) Renal arteriogram.

Discussion

The mechanism of production of the hypertension is as follows: the stenosis produces ischaemic change in the right kidney leading to the production of increased plasma renin. Raised plasma renin converts increased amounts of angiotensinogen to angiotensin I which is then converted to angiotensin II. This has a marked direct pressor effect and also acts on the zona glomerulosa of the adrenals to produce aldosterone. Aldosterone produces a pressor effect by increasing sodium and water reabsorption from the collecting ducts of the nephron.

This patient demonstrates hypokalaemic alkalosis with raised plasma renin activity. The latter excludes primary hyperaldosteronism. In addition the hypokalaemia would be more marked in primary hyperaldoteronism.

The plasma renin activity is greater on the right but also raised on the left, indicating secondary renal ischaemia on that side.

Renal arteriography is essential to delineate the site of the lesion as a guide for operative management. Currently, percutaneous transluminal angioplasty is used in some centres.

Beta blockers suppress plasma renin activity and therefore their use is logical but other agents may be needed. Angiotensin converting enzyme inhibitors, such as captopril, are known to cause reversible acute renal failure in some cases of right renal artery stenosis.

Further reading

FORFAR, p. 1069
GABRIEL, R. (1985) *Postgraduate Nephrology*, 3rd edn. London: Butterworths
NELSON, p. 212, 1380, 1490

Answer 13

(1) Macrocytic anaemia.
    Vitamin B_{12} deficiency.
    Terminal ileal disease.
(2) Crohn's disease.

Discussion

The Schilling test is a means of assessing vitamin B_{12} absorption. A small dose of ^{57}Co- or ^{60}Co-labelled vitamin B_{12} is given orally followed by injection of a large 'flushing' dose of unlabelled vitamin. In normal individuals, 10–30% of the labelled vitamin is subsequently excreted. In pernicious anaemia less than 3% appears in the urine but this returns to normal levels if the test is repeated with exogenous intrinsic factor (IF). If, however, malabsorption is from disease of the terminal ileum (where vitamin B_{12} is absorbed), there will be no increase in urine excretion of labelled vitamin B_{12} with intrinsic factor. (An alternative method involves using a dual isotope, [^{58}Co]vitamin B_{12} and [^{57}Co]vitamin B_{12} bound to IF.)

Crohn's disease is the most likely cause of this boy's malabsorption, and would also explain his short stature and abdominal pain. His serum iron and folate levels are within normal limits, indicating that the malabsorption is not generalized. Vitamin B_{12} absorption often remains adequate in Crohn's disease until the development of either a fistula with bacterial overgrowth, obstruction or following resection. Ulcerative colitis may affect the ileum but is unlikely to present without diarrhoea. Crohn's disease has a more insidious onset and may present without any obvious abdominal symptoms. Tuberculosis of the ileum is rare in the UK except in immigrants, but may cause specific vitamin B_{12} malabsorption. Resection of the terminal ileum for whatever cause, or bacterial overgrowth in the blind loop syndrome may also cause similar effects. Even rarer causes of vitamin B_{12} malabsorption include the Immerslund–Grasbeck syndrome, an autosomal recessive condition associated with unexplained proteinuria, and transcobalamin II deficiency, the carrier protein for vitamin B_{12}. Neither of these conditions would present in this manner. Barium studies would help to substantiate the diagnosis.

Further reading

MERRICK, M. V. (1980) Nuclear and sonic diagnostic methods. In *Scientific Foundations of Gastroenterology*, edited by W. Sircus and A. N. Smith. London: William Heinemann Medical Books Ltd
NELSON, pp. 920–924
TRIPP, J. H. and MULLER, D. P. R. (1984) In *Chemical Pathology in the Sick Child*, edited by B. E. Clayton and J. M. Round, pp. 150–175 Oxford: Blackwell Scientific Publications
WALKER-SMITH, J. A., HAMILTON, J. R. and WALKER, W. A. (1983) Inflammatory and related diseases. In *Practical Paediatric Gastroenterology*, pp. 268–296. London: Butterworths

Answer 14

(1) Turner's syndrome (XO).
(2) Oedema of the neck and feet.
    Horseshoe kidneys.

Discussion

(1) The chromosome picture shows an absence of one X- chromosome, i.e. Turner's syndrome.
(2) Turner's syndrome occurs in 1 in 5000 live births, the majority (95%) of such conceptions being aborted spontaneously.

In the neonate, oedema of the hands and feet may be noted (Bonnevie–Ullrich syndrome) and webbing of the neck is the result of soft tissue oedema in that region while *in utero*. The infants are often of low birth weight.

Other major morphological features include:

Short stature (later in life)
Pigmented naevi (later in life) 60%
High palate 45%
Short neck 71%
Low hair line 73%
Shield chest 60%
Cubitus valgus 58%
Hypoplastic hyperconvex nails 73%
Anomalous auricles 80%

Chromosomal analysis is important to exclude the 45X/46XY mosaic type which, because of the 46XY cell line, predisposes to gonadal neoplasia – thus necessitating surgical removal of the gonads.

Internal organs meriting special investigation include the cardiovascular system (20% have abnormalities of which 70% are coarctation) and the renal system (60% having some structural variations); 50% of Turner's syndrome have a perceptual hearing loss.

The mean IQ is 95; 20% have a degree of mental retardation and often their performance scores are below verbal scores. Endocrine problems are discussed elsewhere.

Further reading

FORFAR, pp. 918, 1137
NELSON, pp. 307, 1501
SMITH, D. W. (1982) In *Recognisable patterns of Human Malformation*, edited by D. W. Smith and K. L. Jones, pp. 72–75. Philadelphia: W. B. Saunders

Answer 15

(1) Transient growth delay.
    Partial growth hormone deficiency.
(2) Repeat insulin test after androgen priming.

Discussion

The insulin stress test shows a partial deficiency in growth hormone (hGH) secretion (peak levels >7 but <15 mIU/l). Thyroid function is normal. In the majority of boys presenting at or near adolescence with short stature and relatively slow growth velocity, this response is due to transient growth hormone deficiency. Growth hormone production returns to normal when puberty becomes fully established. True growth hormone deficiency can present in the same way and there is probably a wide overlap between these two groups. Growth hormone provocation tests should be repeated after androgen priming in boys or after oestrogen priming in girls (in whom the condition is much rarer); in transient deficiency growth hormone production should then be normal.

Further reading

PREECE, M. A. (1981) Growth hormone deficiency. In *Clinical Paediatric Endocrinology*, edited by C. G. D. Brook, pp. 285–304. Oxford: Blackwell Scientific Publications

Answer 16

Wiskott–Aldrich syndrome.

Discussion

Wiskott–Aldrich syndrome is a sex-linked recessive disorder characterized by thrombocytopenia, eczema and immunodeficiency. Characteristically, IgA and IgE are increased but IgM decreased. There may also be a lymphopenia. Patients have abnormalities of platelet aggregation, defective T-cell function and produce a particularly poor antibody response to polysaccharide antigens.

The presentation is usually within the first 6 months of life with an episode of bleeding such as melaena, haematemesis, bruising or haematuria. The immunological abnormalities become more severe with increasing age. Children have increased susceptibility to both bacterial and viral infections and commonly have recurrent episodes of otitis media and pneumonia. The mortality is high with few patients surviving into their teens. A majority die from infection, but bleeding, particularly intraventricular haemorrhage, is also a common cause of death. Those children that survive longer are at increased risk of developing lymphoreticular malignancies.

Transfer factor has been used in Wiskott–Aldrich syndrome but without evidence of any increase in patient survival. Tissue-matched bone marrow transplantation is the only effective treatment. Splenectomy, although increasing platelet numbers and improving function, increases the susceptibility to infection even further.

Selective IgM deficiency can occur either as a rare primary disorder or more commonly in adults secondary to lymphomas. Atopic eczema is associated with a raised IgE but not with low IgM or thrombocytopenia.

Further reading

HAYWARD, A. R. (1983) Specific immunodeficiency. In *Paediatric Immunology*, edited by J. F. Soothill, A. R. Hayward and C. B. S. Wood, pp. 156–211. Oxford: Blackwell Scientific Publications

Answer 17

(1) The EEG shows slow wave activity of increased amplitude over the left frontal region (leads 1 + 2 + 5).
(2) Left frontal region.
(3) A tumour or abscess.

Discussion

Generalized slowing is seen with sedation, encephalitis and encephalopathy. Local slowing with high amplitude waves is seen with local space-occupying lesions.

This child would need a computerized tomographic (CT) scan to define the lesion.

Answer 18

(1) Glanzmann's disease.
(2) Yes.

Discussion

The older girl has Glanzmann's disease. This is a functional disorder of platelets leading to a prolonged bleeding time.

The platelets are of normal size, unlike Bernard–Soulier disease in which platelets are abnormally large. There is also a condition of familial microcytic platelets.

Glanzmann's disease is inherited in an autosomal recessive manner so her younger sister has a 1:4 chance of the same disorder.

Further reading

WILLOUGHBY, M. L. N. (1977) *Paediatric Hematology*, p. 293. Edinburgh: Churchill

Answer 19

(1) A wide air–bone gap.
(2) A conductive hearing loss.
(3) Serous otitis media.

Discussion

The symbols [and] represent bone conduction, and the symbols O and X represent air conduction on the right and left, respectively.

In this case only the audiogram from the right side is shown. There is an auditory loss of around 40 dB and normal bone conduction. The latter implies a normal neurosensory pathway, and so the impairment must lie in the middle ear.

Further reading

FORFAR, p. 1717

Answer 20

(1) First degree heart block.
    Incomplete right bundle-branch block.
(2) Left-to-right shunt at atrial level.
(3) Ostium secundum atrial septal defect (ASD).

Discussion

The ECG shows a sinus rhythm of 100 beats/min. The P waves are normal but the P–R interval of 0.18 seconds is prolonged (upper limit of normal for age and heart rate 0.16 s). A prolonged P–R interval without dropped beats fulfils the criteria for first degree heart block. The QRS duration is 0.08 seconds, i.e. at the upper limit of normal for age. There is an rsR' or rSR' pattern in the right ventricular leads V4R and V1 and slurred S waves in the left ventricular leads 1, AVL, V4 and V6. These QRS changes are characteristic of a right bundle-branch block, but this is termed 'incomplete' as the QRS duration is not prolonged.

The catheter data show significant step-up in oxygen saturation in the right atrium, indicative of a left-to-right shunt at atrial level. This can occur with an atrial septal defect or anomalous pulmonary venous drainage, the latter being rare. The right ventricular pressure is slightly raised and there is a gradient of 12 mmHg across the pulmonary valve. This gradient is probably due to increased flow rather than due to anatomical pulmonary stenosis. True pulmonary stenosis should be suspected with gradients >20 mmHg.

Cardiac catheterization is not usually necessary for making the diagnosis of an atrial septal defect, as the clinical, ECG, X-ray, and echo findings are usually sufficient, and it is only undertaken if other abnormalities are suspected. An ostium primum defect may show similar haemodynamic changes on catheterization, but in such a case there would be left axis deviation on ECG and it would be easily distinguishable on echo. Left ventricular angiography is usually diagnostic in ostium primum defects showing mitral regurgitation and left ventricular outflow obstruction.

Further reading

FOX, K. M. (1980) Atrial septal defects. In *Heart Disease in Infancy and Children*, edited by G. Graham and E. Rossi, pp. 233–245. London: Edward Arnold
JORDON, S. C. and SCOTT, O. (1981) *Heart Disease in Paediatrics*, 2nd edn, pp. 93–108. London: Butterworths
PARK, M. K. and GUNTHEROTH, W. G. (1981) *How to Read Pediatric ECGs*. Chicago: Year Book Medical Publishers Inc.

Answer 21

(1) Normal glomerular and tubular function.
(2) Psychogenic polydipsia.

Discussion

In this child the differential diagnosis for polyuria/polydipsia without glycosuria is three-fold – diabetes insipidus, chronic renal failure and psychogenic polydipsia. Concentrating activity is also impaired in hypercalcaemia and hypokalaemia.

Chronic renal failure can usually be excluded knowing urea, creatinine or creatinine clearance results.

The differentiation of diabetes insipidus (either central or nephrogenic) and psychogenic polydipsia can be difficult because prolonged polydipsia may lead to impaired concentrating ability, as in this child. Normally, after a water deprivation test, a urine osmolality of >800 mosmol/kg would be expected. In diabetes insipidus it would be <200 mosmol/kg.

A water deprivation test is potentially dangerous in the child who cannot concentrate his/her urine and should therefore be carefully supervised with serial observations (heart rate, respiratory rate, and blood pressure) with osmolality urea and electrolyte measurements when indicated. These children may rapidly become dehydrated.

This child's estimated serum osmolality ($2[Na^+ + K^+]$ + glucose + urea) is normal (glucose is not significantly raised since there is no glycosuria) – suggesting psychogenic polydipsia rather than polyuria of a pathological nature.

Further reading

NELSON, p. 1437

Answer 22

(1) Hyperkalaemic acidosis.
(2) Renal failure.
(3) Uric acid : creatinine ratio or plasma urate.
(4) Yes – allopurinol and fluids.

Discussion

The patient has developed urate nephropathy or the tumour lysis syndrome.

Tumour lysis syndrome results from the rapid destruction of tumour cells by intensive chemotherapy. These effects include:

(1) Hyperuricaemia.
(2) Hyperphosphataemia.
(3) Hypocalcaemia (unlike other causes of acute renal failure in which it is usually normal).
(4) Hyperkalaemia.
(5) Raised creatinine and urea but not necessarily to renal failure levels.

The uric acid level will be disproportionately higher than the rise in creatinine. The urine uric acid : creatinine ratio is therefore raised. Renal failure will follow if left untreated.

In all cases of newly diagnosed renal failure it is important to exclude obstruction of the urinary tract so an abdominal ultrasound examination is indicated. Leukaemic infiltration could produce the obstruction.

Prevention is possible if allopurinol is commenced before chemotherapy, and continued until the white cell count is normal. Ample fluids should be given throughout. If urate nephropathy occurs, early intervention with high fluid intake, forced alkaline diuresis and allopurinol will normally reverse the biochemical changes. In more severe cases haemodialysis may be required.

Further reading

NELSON, p. 1377

Answer 23

(1) The reducing sugars, i.e. fructose, lactose, galactose, pentoses.
    Salicylates.
    Homogentisic acid.
    Phenothiazines.
(2) Sugar electophoresis or chromatography.
    Ferric chloride test (Phenistix) – phenothiazines will also change ferric chloride to purple.
    Nitroprusside test.
    Toxicology.

(3) Clinistix.
Labstix.
Haemocombistix.
Are all specific for glucose, each using a glucose oxidase test.

Discussion

This question appears quite frequently and, while sideroom testing of urine is not part of everyday clinical practice, a knowledge of this area is still expected.

Further reading

ZILVA, J. F. and PANNALL, P. R. (Eds.) (1979) *Clinical Chemistry in Diagnosis and Treatment*, 3rd edn., p. 207. London: Lloyd-Luke

Answer 24

(1) Conjugated hyperbilirubinaemia.
(2) Neonatal hepatitis and biliary atresia.
(3) Rose bengal excretion test or other isotope excretion tests.
24-hour duodenal aspiration.
Liver biopsy.

Discussion

Direct bilirubin estimation reflects the water-soluble component, i.e. the conjugated component. Extraction with alcohol, i.e. indirect, reflects the unconjugated component.

The differentiation between obstructive jaundice and hepatitis (which, due to inflammation, causes bile duct compression and so partial obstruction) can be difficult, but it is important as the outcome from operative procedures is enhanced by early diagnosis and intervention. Conversely, surgical procedures may worsen hepatitis.

The two conditions may represent the same process (inflammation) occurring at two sites (the intraheptic and extrahepatic biliary tract) with a spectrum of severity in between. Indeed there are documented cases where neonatal hepatitis has progressed to biliary atresia. Often no aetiology is found but there are a number of causes which need to be considered – TORCH infections, *Listeria*, genetic–metabolic problems, e.g. galactosaemia (*see* Forfar, *Table 11.22*, for a complete list).

The clinically important decision is whether to operate; the rose bengal test in theory is useful – less than 10% of the radioisotope should be excreted into the stools in biliary atresia. However, sample collection over a 72-hour period is a problem in the newborn period.

A duodenal tube constantly or intermittently aspirated over a 48-hour period may be useful – if bile is seen then the tract is presumed to be at least partly patent. If bile is not seen, the test must be repeated as occasionally hepatic inflammation is so severe that bile does not escape into the tract despite a patent duct system.

Liver biopsy requires skilled interpretation – in hepatitis there is diffuse giant cell transformation of hepatocytes with necrosis and a cellular infiltrate. In biliary atresia the ducts are small and surrounded by chronic inflammatory elements and bile salt pigments, i.e. the aftermath of sclerosing cholangitis.

Further reading

FORFAR, pp. 183, 505
NELSON, p. 967

Answer 25

(1) Tuberculous meningitis.
(2) Ziehl–Nielsen staining of CSF deposit.
    Chest X-ray.
(3) Quadruple antituberculous therapy.

Discussion

The onset of tuberculous meningitis is usually slow and neurological signs develop as the CSF protein rises.

The CSF findings are classical – the white cell count is rarely above 300, the glucose is low. These findings do not fit with a viral illness and so the absence of organisms on Gram stain requires further investigation. Initially Ziehl–Nielsen staining may reveal the organisms; in the longer term, culture on Loewenstein–Jensen medium is required and sensitivities need to be examined.

The Mantoux test may be negative in the early stages and so a chest X-ray is generally helpful.

All the family members and close friends will need to be investigated until the source is found.

Management would need to be discussed with the microbiologists involved, but it is generally accepted that quadruple therapy is initiated until sensitivities of the organism are available. This includes streptomycin (possibly intrathecally to start with), rifampicin, isoniazide and ethambutol. If the child is vomiting, parenteral streptomycin and isoniazid would be the initial choice.

Further reading

FORFAR, p. 1401
NELSON, p. 716

Answer 26

(1) Intravenous infusion of 0.9% saline with glucose.
Hydrocortisone.
A mineralocorticoid (aldosterone or deoxycorticosterone).
(2) Congenital adrenal hyperplasia.

Discussion

This infant is suffering from a salt-losing crisis. A low serum sodium combined with a high potassium suggests either acute renal failure, as may occur with posterior urethral valves, or adrenal cortical failure. In the former urinary sodium will be low (<20 mmol/l), whereas as in this case urinay sodium loss is marked.

A salt-losing state in an infant of this age, combined with a high potassium, is most likely to be due to congenital adrenal hyperplasia – this has an occurrence of approximately 1 in 5000 live births and in >90% the 21-hydroxylase enzyme is defective. Only a proportion of these infants have significant salt loss. This child shows signs of increased virilization, although often male infants appear normal. Unless urinary sodium is checked the diagnosis may be missed.

Confirmation is made by finding raised plasma 17α-hydroxyprogesterone (samples should be taken after the first 24 hours of birth), and urinary steroid metabolites. ACTH levels are also raised. In 21-hydroxylase deficiency, urinary 17-oxosteroids, 17-oxogenic steroids, 17-hydroxycorticosteroids and pregnanetriol are raised. The 11-oxygenation index (the ratio of 11-hydroxysteroids to 11-deoxysteroids) is also increased. Normal pregnanetriol levels in the first month of life do not exclude 21-hydroxylase deficiency, and this investigation is now being superseded by radioimmunoassay of plasma hormones. Salt loss also occurs in the far rarer 20,22-desmolase deficiency, and in 3β-hydroxysteroid dehydrogenase deficiency.

Congenital adrenal hypoplasia, either as an isolated disorder or associated with anencephaly, is a further cause of salt loss.

In the acute management of these children, making the exact diagnosis is of secondary importance. Immediate resuscitation with saline and steroids is required. Salt loss may be very high and babies may require up to 5 g of sodium a day. Hydrocortisone should be combined with a mineralocorticoid. Hypoglycaemia is common and must be treated.

Further reading

BROOK, C. G. D. (1981) Congenital adrenal hyperplasia. In *Clinical Paediatric Endocrinology*, edited by C. G. D. Brook, pp. 453–464. Oxford: Blackwell Scientific Publications

DILLON, M. J. (1981) Salt-losing states. In *Clinical Paediatric Endocrinology*, edited by C. G. D. Brook, pp. 465–478. Oxford: Blackwell Scientific Publications

Answer 27

(1) Alveolar capillary block.
(2) Oedema.
    Infiltration.
    Inflammation/fibrosis.
    Alveolar proteinoses.
    Lymphangiectasis.
    Haemosiderosis

Discussion

The total lung capacity, forced vital capacity, forced expiratory volume in one second, and peak expiratory flow rate are all normal for a child of this age.

The only abnormality is the reduced diffusion capacity which reflects a widened alveolar–capillary space.

This question does not give an adequate history or duration and therefore these figures have to be taken at 'face value' and a differential diagnosis constructed.

None of these conditions are common in childhood.

Oedema may be secondary to cardiac failure or toxic gas inhalation.

Infiltrations are very rare but include malignancies, sarcoid and collagen disorders.

Any inflammatory process may initially present with these findings – some progress to fibrosis, resulting in a restrictive pattern of lung function tests. Examples are post-chemotherapy, post-irradiation and idiopathic (Hamman–Rich).

Further reading

FORFAR, p. 532
NELSON, pp. 1062–1063

Answer 28

(1) Hyponatraemic dehydration.
(2) Prerenal failure.

Discussion

Clinically this child is between 5 and 10% dehydrated and has a plasma sodium of <130 mmol/l. The diagnosis is therefore that of hyponatraemic dehydration, i.e. sodium deficit is greater than that of water. The evidence that this is complicated by prerenal failure is as follows:

(1) Oliguria; renal output <1 ml/kg per h.
(2) Low urinary sodium of <10 mmol/l.

(3) Urine : plasma (U : P) urea ratio >5.
(4) U : P osmolality ratio of >1.3. Plasma osmolality is estimated by 2 × (Na^+ + K^+) + glucose + urea.

These changes may be regarded as physiological. At this stage the kidneys are functioning to retain sodium and to conserve fluid. If losses continue and treatment is not given, then the ability to do this will be outstripped.

In established renal failure urine output is likely to be <0.3 ml/kg per h, urinary sodium >40 mmol/l, U : P urea <5 and U : P osmolality <1.1.

Further reading

GABRIEL R. (1985) *Postgraduate Nephrology,* 3rd edn. London: Butterworths
NELSON, pp. 1357–1361

Answer 29

(1) Haemolytic anaemia.
(2) Infective.
    Autoimmune.
    Malignant.
(3) Antibody titres or Monospot test.
    Antinuclear antibodies.
    Lymph node biopsy.

Discussion

The red cell changes are characteristic of all forms of haemolytic anaemia – spherocytes are small red cells which have lost their biconcave shape as a result of the pathological process. Spherocytes have a shortened life as they are more sensitive to lysis and sequestration in the spleen.

The reticulocytosis indicates marrow compensation for haemolysis; where the demand is great normoblasts may be seen in the peripheral circulation.

Urobilinogen is derived from stercobilin which has been reabsorbed from the bowel and excreted in the urine. It is a non-quantitative test, but a useful indicator of haemolysis.

The absence of haemoglobulin from the urine excludes disseminated intravascular coagulation, haemolytic uraemic syndrome and paroxysmal nocturnal haemoglobinuria.

The recent onset, and lymphadenopathy, make inherited forms of haemolytic anaemia unlikely.

The three groups of pathological process would therefore be:

(1) Infective, e.g. infectious mononucleosis, cytomegalovirus.
(2) Autoimmune, e.g. systemic lupus erythematosus.
(3) Malignant, e.g. reticulosis.

Autoantibodies are often useful to differentiate viral or mycoplasma infections (which produce cold antibodies) from systemic lupus erythematosus or reticuloses (which produce warm antibodies), but are not diagnostic of any one pathological process. Likewise a positive Coombs' test is very useful but not diagnostic.

Further reading

FORFAR, pp. 945, 956
NELSON, p. 1230

Answer 30

Right bundle-branch block.

Discussion

The ECG shows the following characteristic features of right bundle-branch block (RBBB):
(1) A prolonged QRS duration (approximately 0.1 s with an upper limit of normal for age of 0.06 s).
(2) Terminal slurring of the QRS complex directed to the right (slurred S in I and V6, and slurred R in aVR) and anteriorly (slurred R in V4R, V1–V4).
(3) Right axis deviation (approximately +120 with upper limit of normal for age <110).
(4) ST depression and T wave inversion over the blocked ventricle (V4R–V4).

Right bundle-branch block is one of the more common conduction disturbances in children. In many cases it is due to right ventricular volume overload (e.g. ostium secundum atrial septal defect) with the normal conduction pathway considerably increased in length. In such children, the QRS duration is usually only slightly increased, and is therefore sometimes termed 'incomplete right bundle-branch block'. Actual damage to the conduction fibres can occur after open heart surgery involving ventriculotomy, as in this child. The main right bundle itself is usually not affected but right bundle-branch block follows the disruption of the subendothelial Purkinje fibres of the right ventricle. It should be remembered that voltage criteria from the ECG cannot be used to make a diagnosis of ventricular hypertrophy when bundle-branch block is present, as the ventricular forces are asynchronous and may be unopposed.

Further reading

HARRIS, L. C. and FEINSTEIN, E. (1979) *Understanding ECGs in Infants and Children*, 2nd edn. Boston: Little, Brown and Company
PARK, M. K. and GUNTHEROTH, W. G. (1981) *How to Read Pediatric ECGs*. Chicago: Year Book Medical Publishers Inc.

Answer 31

(1) Congenital chloridorrhoea.
(2) Potassium chloride supplements.

Discussion

This child has an extremely low plasma chloride and potassium with a high plasma bicarbonate. Urinary chloride is undetectable whereas stool chloride loss is very high. This is diagnostic of congenital chloridorrhoea (also known as 'congenital alkalosis with diarrhoea' or 'familial chloride diarrhoea').

This rare familial disorder is due to a failure of active chloride absorption in the ileum and possibly also in the colon. Passive absorption with exchange of chloride for bicarbonate ions can occur. Sodium transport is not affected. Chronic diarrhoea is caused by the osmotic effect of the unabsorbed chloride ions and there are secondary losses of sodium and potassium ions.

Children with this condition are often premature, and develop hyperbilirubinaemia. Although diarrhoea is usually noted in the first weeks, some infants may not present until later with severe dehydration. Growth and motor development are retarded. Chronic water and electrolyte deficit leads to secondary hyperaldosteronism with subsequent high urinary potassium and hydrogen ion loss, causing hypokalaemic alkalosis.

The diagnosis is confirmed by measuring faecal electrolytes. In the first month the chloride concentration is from 50 to 150 mmol/l, but subsequently remains between 110 and 180 mmol/l (normal range 6–17 mmol/l). The urinary chloride is undetectable.

Treatment consists of giving KCl in quantities sufficient to maintain normal plasma electrolytes and acid–base balance. The prognosis is variable; some children die in infancy, others may have a normal lifespan.

Further reading

HARRIES, J. T. (1977) *Essentials of Paediatric Gastroenterology*, pp. 206–208. Edinburgh: Churchill Livingstone
WALKER-SMITH, J. A., HAMILTON, J. R. and WALKER, W. A. (1983) *Practical Paediatric Gastroenterology*, p. 263. London: Butterworths

Answer 32

(1) Isolated growth hormone deficiency.
(2) Thrice weekly growth hormone injections.

Discussion

This child is below the 3rd centile for height, his growth velocity over the previous 12 months has been below the 10th centile. He is relatively obese with an increased skin-fold thickness and his bone age is significantly reduced.

On investigation, he has severe growth hormone deficiency (peak level <7 mIU/l, normal response >15 mIU/l) but with no evidence of other pituitary hormone deficiencies. The cortisol response is satisfactory (normal, peak >400 nmol/l). The LHRH shows a normal prepubertal pattern. He therefore has isolated growth hormone deficiency (IGHD), although it is difficult to be certain that there is no deficiency in gonadotrophins until after puberty has occurred.

The aetiology of this condition is often unknown, although slowly enlarging pituitary tumours, not seen on skull X-ray or on lower resolution CT brain scans, may present with isolated growth hormone deficiency. Children with 'idiopathic' isolated growth hormone deficiency should be carefully followed and scanned with the highest resolution machine available. There is also an association with birth trauma in a significant minority of cases of isolated growth hormone deficiency, and occasionally there is a definite hereditary cause.

In the UK, isolated growth hormone deficiency is more common than growth hormone deficiency combined with deficiencies of other pituitary hormones. Partial growth hormone deficiency is also seen and this is nearly always as an isolated deficiency.

Growth hormone deficiency may be due to developmental anomalies, such as malformation of midline brain structures, intracranial space-occupying lesions, cranial irradiation or secondary to infection. It has also been reported in congenital rubella, mitochondrial myopathy, Fanconi's anaemia, ataxia telangiectasia, Bloom's syndrome, Turner's syndrome and Russell–Silver dwarfism (although in the last two in the great majority of patients growth hormone production is normal and is not the cause of short stature).

Treatment for growth hormone deficiency consists of injections with methionine-hGH (biosynthetic growth hormone) three times a week. Previously, growth hormone was extracted from human pituitary glands (the hormone is species specific), but this was withdrawn in the UK and the USA in 1985 after three deaths from Creutzfeldt–Jakob disease were reported from the USA in young adults who had been treated with hGH in the 1960s and 1970s. One further case was reported in the UK in 1985.

Other endocrine disorders, primarily hypothyroidism and Cushing's syndrome, are often associated with short stature. Growth hormone response may be reduced on provocation testing. These should be repeated after treatment of the primary condition. In Laron dwarfism (somatomedin deficiency) the clinical picture may be identical to growth hormone deficiency, but growth hormone levels are high.

Non-endocrine disease may also present as short stature, particularly coeliac and Crohn's disease, even in the absence of abdominal symptoms.

Further reading

PREECE, M. A. (1981) Growth hormone deficiency. In *Clinical Paediatric Endocrinology*, edited by C. G. D. Brook, pp. 285–304. Oxford: Blackwell Scientific Publications

TANNER, J. M. (1984) Growth and its problems. In *Chemical Pathology in the Sick Child*, edited by B. E. Clayton and J. M. Round, pp. 296–311. Oxford: Blackwell Scientific Publications

Answer 33

(1) Cystinuria.
(2) Ornithine, arginine, lysine and cystine.
(3) High fluid intake.
   Sodium bicarbonate to form alkaline urine.
   D-Penicillamine.
   Surgical intervention for large stones.

Discussion

Cystinuria is caused by a defect in the proximal renal and intestinal transport of lysine, arginine, and ornithine and cystine. Blood levels of these amino acids are normal. Inheritance is autosomal recessive. Lysine, arginine and ornithine are readily soluble but cystine forms crystals in acid urine. These crystals have a characteristic hexagonal pattern and 'maple sugar' appearance (not smell!). Bilateral, multiple radio-opaque calculi, which may be 'stag-horn', form in a minority of those with cystinuria. Presentation, usually in the second or third decade, is with ureteric colic or obstruction.

The urine cyanide–nitroprusside test is positive in the presence of disulphides and therefore positive in cystinuria, homocystinuria, generalized aminoaciduria, Fanconi's syndrome, β-mercapto-lactate-cysteine disulphiduria and sulphite–oxidase deficiency. However, the combination with renal calculi is strongly suggestive of cystinuria. Although still performed routinely in many hospitals, a number of laboratories have discontinued this test in view of the toxicity of the reagents.

Treatment consists of increasing fluid intake to maintain a urinary output of at least 4 litres a day and maintaining the urine at pH 8 (at which point cystine becomes very soluble) by giving large amounts of sodium bicarbonate. Both of these are difficult to achieve in practice and it is often necessary to give D-penicillamine. Large stones may require surgical management although open surgical removal is rarely indicated.

Further reading

FORFAR, p. 1021
NELSON, pp. 430, 1349
SEGALS, S. and THIER, S. L. (1983) Cystinuria. In *The Metabolic Basis of Inherited Diseases,* edited by J. B. Stanbury, J. B. Wyngaarden, D. S. Fredrickson, J. L. Goldstein and M. S. Brown, pp. 1774–1791. New York: McGraw-Hill Book Company

Answer 34

(1) Combined metabolic and respiratory acidosis.
(2) Oxygen therapy.
(3) Respiratory distress syndrome.

Discussion

The pH is low – a combined effect from a high Pco_2 and a low bicarbonate (the base excess directly reflects the bicarbonate).

The Po_2 is maintained in the normal range by the use of high concentration headbox oxygen. This infant requires ventilation to control the CO_2 retention. The metabolic component could be managed with either volume expansion or a bicarbonate infusion.

The gestation of the infant is not mentioned – but the commonest cause for this picture would be respiratory distress syndrome in the pre-term infant. (If the question had stated a term infant then an aspiration syndrome would be the more common aetiology.)

Further reading

ROBERTON, N. R. C. (1981) *A Manual of Neonatal Intensive Care.* London: Edward Arnold

Answer 35

(1) Treat raised intracranial pressure.
   Establish diuresis.
   Give chelating agents (dimercaprol, calcium disodium ethylenediamine tetraacetate (edetate)).
(2) Lead encephalopathy.

Discussion

This boy has severe lead poisoning: blood lead levels are normally less than 1.4 µmol/l and those above 4 µmol/l are associated with a high risk of encephalopathy. Lead inhibits several of the enzymes involved in haem synthesis; chronic exposure leads to a microcytic hypochromic anaemia, raised urinary δ-aminolaevulinic acid and coproporphyrin. Free erythrocyte protoporphyrin is also raised. Other evidence of chronic exposure includes basophilic stippling of red cells, generalized aminoaciduria and glycosuria and 'lead lines' at the metaphysis of long bones on X-ray. If lead had been ingested recently, there might also be radio-opaque bodies seen on abdominal X-rays. Urinary δ-aminolaevulinic acid is raised in acute intermittent porphyria but this is also associated with increased excretion of porphobilinogen which is not found in lead poisoning.

Urgent treatment is necessary. Mannitol may be used to reduce intracranial pressure and to establish a diuresis before starting chelation therapy. Gastric lavage with sodium sulphate or magnesium sulphate will remove any lead still present in the stomach. Chelation with dimercaprol (British anti-Lewisite, BAL) given intramuscularly combined with calcium disodium ethylenediamine tetraacetate (Ca EDTA), intramuscularly or intravenously, should be given over a period of several days. Lead poisoning of this severity has a high mortality. In milder cases and in the recovery phase from more severe poisoning, D-penicillamine given orally is an effective chelating agent, but should only be used if there is no possibility of continuing exposure.

Further reading

FORFAR, pp. 1776–1803
NELSON, pp. 1800–1803
SHELLSHEAR, I. (1979) Acute lead poisoning. In *Paediatric Emergencies,* edited by J. A. Black, pp. 369–372. London: Butterworths

Answer 36

(1) Klinefelter's syndrome.
(2) One in 500 although there are, like other trisomies, higher risks with advancing maternal age.
(3) Almost nil – generally people with Klinefelter's syndrome are sterile, but one or two offspring have been reported in the literature.

Answer 37

(1) Under-treatment of asthma.
    Pneumothorax.
(2) Humidified 40% oxygen.
    Inhaled nebulized salbutamol.

Discussion

The diagnosis of pneumothorax can easily be overlooked on clinical examination of a child whose chest is overinflated and has reduced air entry. A clinical pointer to this diagnosis would be pain on the affected side and if suspected a chest X-ray should be obtained immediately.

It must not be forgotten that oxygen is an important line of therapy in acute asthma – hypoxic patients have considerable sympathetic output which further aggravates the anxiety already present.

Inhaled salbutamol is preferred for ease of administration and low incidence of side-effects compared to intravenous salbutamol.

Failure to respond to inhaled treatment would be an indication for intravenous aminophylline and for hydrocortisone.

If a clinically significant pneumothorax were present it would require drainage.

Answer 38

(1) Type I pauciarticular juvenile chronic arthritis.
(2) Analgesic nephropathy.
    Amyloid.
(3) Slit lamp examination for chronic iridocyclitis.

Discussion

There is plenty of scope for questions around the classification of juvenile chronic arthritis. This girl has fewer than four joints affected; the disease has been present for many years, starting in early childhood, so her clinical classification is therefore in the type I pauciarticular group.

These children are rheumatoid factor negative but about half have antinuclear antibodies. There is an association with HLA-DR5 and -DR8. This form of disease is not usually found in adults and ocular damage secondary to chronic iridocyclitis occurs in about 10%; one or both eyes may be affected and its severity is not related to the severity of the arthritis. Likewise it may occur without the usual signs of redness, reduced visual acuity, pain and photosensitivity.

Slit lamp examination is recommended three or four times a year to detect the increased cell and protein content of the anterior chamber of the eye.

Amyloid occurs in about 5% of children with juvenile chronic arthritis in Europe. It is a secondary form of amyloid with deposition mainly in kidneys, spleen, liver and adrenals of AA type amyloid – a molecule derived from the larger SAA precursor by proteolysis. Its extracellular deposition causes damage by compression and disruption of the glomeruli, resulting in proteinuria and haematuria.

Analgesic nephropathy is seen less today as more powerful non-steroidal and safer anti-inflammatory agents are available.

Further reading

NELSON, pp. 564, 1773

Answer 39

(1) Reduce calories, phosphorus and sodium.
(2) Hypernatraemic dehydration.
    Hypocalcaemic convulsions.
(3) Cow's milk plus sugar.

Discussion

	Breast milk	Cow's milk	Modified milk
Calories (g/100 ml)	70	67	65
Protein (g/100 ml)	1.1	3.3	1.6
Fat (g/100 ml)	4.2	3.7	3.3
Sodium (mg/100 ml)	15	52	21
Potassium (mg/100 ml)	60	140	70
Calcium (mg/100 ml)	35	120	55
Phosphorus (mg/100 ml)	15	98	49

The table is self-explanatory. Some knowledge of the constituents of breast and bottle formulae is expected. Obesity could reasonably be included as a clinical complication of using the formula.

SI units are given in the question in parentheses as mg/100 ml is still used for milk products!

Further reading

FORFAR, p. 1922

Answer 40

Left atrial hypertrophy (LAH).

Discussion

The P wave represents the depolarization of both atria with right atrial depolarization occurring first. It is often best seen in II, V1 and V2. P duration is normally 0.06±0.02 s in children, but if it exceeds 0.1 second, in any lead, it is diagnostic of left atrial hypertrophy. Left atrial hypertrophy is best seen in V1 where there is terminal P wave inversion. In the limb leads the P wave appears broad and notched. With right atrial hypertrophy the P wave duration is normal but P amplitude is increased (usually seen best in lead II). In biatrial hypertrophy there is a combination of both increased P wave duration and amplitude. Unlike the change in QRS axis that occurs in ventricular hypertrophy, the P axis is not affected by atrial hypertrophy.

In this ECG there is a sinus rhythm of 63 beats/min, the P–R interval is 0.12 s, the P wave is bifid and prolonged, and the P amplitude is 1 mm (upper limit of normal 3 mm). Left atrial hypertrophy is therefore present. A sinus rate of 63 beats/min is not abnormal at this age.

Further reading

HARRIS, L. C. and FEINSTEIN, E. (1979) *Understanding ECGs in Infants and Children*, 2nd edn. Boston: Little, Brown and Company

PARK, M. K. and GUNTHEROTH, W. G. (1981) *How to Read Pediatric ECGs*. Chicago: Year Book Medical Publishers Inc.

Answer 41

Diabetes mellitus.

Discussion

Glycosuria may be present in a number of conditions, particularly in renal disease, but there are few disorders that present in this manner. Acute pancreatitis, CNS tumours or infection, Cushing's syndrome, phaeochromocytoma, and glucocorticoid treatment may all cause hyperglycaemia, but a child with a history as given in this question almost certainly has diabetes mellitus.

A majority of patients enter a 'honeymoon' period within 2–3 months of the initial diagnosis with exogenous insulin requirements falling to 50% or less of their initial level. Some enter a phase of complete remission, lasting approximately 6 weeks, when insulin can be stopped altogether without inducing hyperglycaemia. During this time endogenous insulin production is sufficient to maintain normal metabolic control. Unfortunately, in all patients insulin requirements will increase, usually within the first 3 months following diagnosis.

There is a true transient diabetes mellitus that occurs rarely in some hypertrophic infants within the first 6 weeks of life. The aetiology is unknown, but thought to be due to a delay in maturity of pancreatic β-cells. Hyperglycaemia is accompanied by relatively low levels of insulin.

The condition lasts a few weeks only, following which glucose tolerance tests return to normal.

Further reading

NELSON, p. 1414
WEBER, B. (1981) Physiological aspects of diabetes mellitus. In *Clinical Paediatric Endocrinology*, edited by C. G. D. Brook, pp. 578–615. Oxford: Blackwell Scientific Publications

Answer 42

(1) Congenital nephrotic syndrome.
(2) Increased amniotic fluid in α-fetoprotein.

Discussion

This neonate is oedematous, with severe hypoalbuminaemia and highly selective proteinuria, and therefore has nephrotic syndrome. Idiopathic (minimal change) nephrotic syndrome is very rare in the first 6 months of life, but congenital syphilis may cause a membranous nephropathy during this time. However, presentation in the first weeks of life (particularly in association with a family history) is almost certainly due to congenital nephrotic syndrome. This is usually an autosomal recessive disorder, most commonly seen in Scandinavia and known as Finnish type congenital nephrotic syndrome. Light microscopy may show normal glomeruli but with cystic dilatation of the proximal tubules. On electron microscopy, there is fusion of the glomerular basement membrane foot processes. α-Fetoprotein is raised during pregnancy, the placenta is abnormally large (>25% birth weight), and infants are usually born prematurely. Presentation is within the first days or weeks after birth. Palliative treatment with diuretics, sodium restriction and γ-globulins may prolong life but death from renal failure within the first 24 months is inevitable. Bilateral nephrectomy, with subsequent dialysis and followed by transplantation, has been attempted with some degree of success.

Other causes of nephrotic syndrome in the newborn include renal vein thrombosis and renal tumours. In these cases the proteinuria would not be selective.

Further reading

FORFAR, pp. 1055–1056
NELSON, p. 1329

Answer 43

(1) Metabolic alkalosis with compensatory hypokalaemia.
(2) Duodenal ulcer leading to pyloric stenosis.
(3) Barium meal or gastroscopy.

Discussion

Peptic ulcers do occur in childhood – duodenal ulcers seem more related to increased acid output (often a strong family history), whereas gastric ulcers seem related to poor tissue resistance, e.g. anoxia, poor perfusion or drugs (steroids/salicylates).

In the pre-school child the presentation is often through poor growth, recurrent vomiting and gastrointestinal haemorrhage, whereas the school-age child presents with the adult picture although the pain is often less specific and eating provides less relief.

Other diagnoses to be considered in a child who is vomiting with recurrent abdominal pain are upper gastrointestinal obstructions, e.g. Ladd's bands, volvulus and other congenital problems.

Where the ulcers are severe and recurrent a raised serum gastrin level would indicate a Zollinger–Ellison syndrome.

The potassium is low as it is exchanged for hydrogen ions in the renal tubule in an attempt to compensate for the loss of hydrogen ions in vomiting.

Further reading

FORFAR, p. 437
NELSON, p. 902

Answer 44

(1) Marrow hypoplasia.
(2) Environmental toxins.
    Marrow infiltration.

Discussion

This child appears normal – thereby making a number of inherited forms associated with congenital defects (Fanconi) unlikely – although a small number do look normal resulting from variable penetrance. Inherited forms not associated with congenital defects have been described (Estren and Dameshek) and there are forms associated with dyskeratosis congenita.

In about half the cases of marrow hypoplasia, no cause is found, but in the remainder the following possibilities need consideration:

(1) Direct toxins – lead, benzenes, etc.
(2) Idiosyncratic toxic response – chloramphenicol, phenobarbitone, phenytoin, sulphonamides and phenylbutazone.
(3) Postinfections – hepatitis, infectious mononucleosis.
(4) Infiltration – leukaemia, osteopetrosis, myelofibrosis.
(5) Postirradiation.
(6) Associated with paroxysmal nocturnal haemoglobinuria.

Further reading

FORFAR, p. 943
NELSON, p. 1233

Answer 45

(1) Oestrogen-secreting ovarian tumour.
(2) Abdominal ultrasound.
    LHRH stimulation test.
(3) Surgical removal.

Discussion

The combination of breast development, vaginal bleeding and a palpable ovary is suggestive of either (1) an oestrogen-secreting ovarian tumour, (2) constitutional (idiopathic) precocious puberty with an ovarian cyst, or (3) a gonadatrophin-secreting tumour with an ovarian cyst. In children, most functioning ovarian lesions are neoplastic, oestrogen secreting and primarily consist of granuloma cells. Non-functioning ovarian cysts are more common than ovarian tumours and those occurring in constitutional precocious puberty (very rare at this age) are likely to be secondary to increased pituitary gonadatrophins. In constitutional precocious puberty and with gonadotrophin-secreting tumours, plasma and urinary oestrogens will not be markedly raised, whereas with oestrogen-secreting tumours both are very high, and an LHRH stimulation test will show normal or low values of LH and follicle-stimulating hormone (FSH).

Granulosa cell tumours may be either malignant or benign. Surgical removal should be undertaken as soon as the diagnosis is made. Following this a withdrawal bleed is common, but subsequently oestrogen levels return to normal and signs of precocious puberty disappear.

Further reading

RAYNER, P. H. W. (1981) Early puberty. In *Clinical Paediatric Endocrinology*, edited by C. G. D. Brook, pp. 224–239. Oxford: Blackwell Scientific Publications

Answer 46

(1) Salicylate poisoning.
(2) Salicylate level.
    Ferric chloride (Gerhardt's) test.

Discussion

This girl has a partially compensated metabolic acidosis and reducing substances in the urine. Clinistix is a specific assay for glucose in which glucose oxidase catalyses the oxidation of glucose to glucuronic acid and hydrogen peroxide. The peroxide then reacts with a chromogen to form a violet colour. Clinitest will also give a positive result with reducing sugars other than glucose, i.e. galactose, lactose, fructose, and pentoses. Lactosuria occurs in hereditary or acquired intestinal lactase deficiency and may also be present in the urine of lactating mothers. Fructosuria is present in hereditary fructosaemia, benign fructosuria, and after ingestion of large quantities of fruit or confectionery. Galactosuria is found in galactosaemia. Pentosuria is associated with some drugs but may also occur after eating large amounts of certain fruits such as grapes. Vitamin C, L-dopa, naladixic acid and probenecid may all give a false positive result in high doses. Homogentisic acid gives a black discoloration with Clinitest. Aspirin is conjugated with glucuronic acid in the liver and then excreted in the urine; glucuronates have reducing properties and will give a positive result if present in substantial amounts.

The diagnosis in a girl of this age is almost certainly salicylate poisoning, although other rare causes (e.g. severe liver disease) might give a similar picture. In salicylate poisoning, hyperventilation may initially cause a respiratory alkalosis but this is followed by the development of a metabolic acidosis. The alkalotic phase is often short lived in children. Ketonuria is often present.

The diagnosis may be confirmed by measuring the serum salicylate level; levels less than 3.0 mmol/l are rarely associated with symptoms, peak levels are reached within 2–3 hours of ingestion. The ferric chloride test is now rarely performed, since salicylate levels are easily obtained. It involves adding 3% ferric chloride dropwise to urine. In the presence of acetoacetate or salicylates a red-purple colour develops. If the urine is then boiled for several minutes ketones are destroyed but the salicylates are unchanged.

Further reading

FORFAR, pp. 1773–1776
NELSON, pp. 1789–1791
SNODGRASS, W. R. (1986) Salicylate toxicity. *Paediatric Clinics of North America*, **33**, 381–391

Answer 47

(1) Vomiting of swallowed maternal blood.
(2) Reassurance.

Discussion

Although the coagulation tests on this infant are prolonged as compared to the (adult) control values, they are all within the normal range for a term infant.

The main differential diagnosis is from haemorrhagic disease of the newborn. This classically presents 24–48 hours after delivery due to a deficiency in vitamin K-dependent coagulation factors (II, VII, IX and X). The prothrombin time (PT) and partial thromboplastin time (PTT) would both be significantly prolonged (PT >20 s, PTT >70 s) while the thrombin time (TT) would be normal. The PT should return to normal within 4 hours of giving vitamin K_1.

The Apt test is a means of differentiating maternal from fetal blood and relies on the fact that HbF is alkali resistant. A specimen of bloody vomit or stool is mixed with water and centrifuged. The supernatant is then mixed with 1% sodium hydroxide solution. If maternal blood is present, HbA is denatured, forming a brownish-yellow colour, fetal blood remaining pink. In this case maternal blood may have been swallowed during delivery or during breast feeding from cracked nipples.

Further reading

FORFAR, pp. 178, 192

Answer 48

(1) Lymphadenitis.. Persistent diarrhoea.
    Skin abscesses. Conjunctivitis.
    Osteomyelitis. Fungal infections.
    Pneumonia. Failure to thrive.
    Bronchitis. Hepatosplenomegaly.
    Dermatitis.
(2) Chronic granulomatous disease.
(3) Antibiotics.
    White cell transfusions.
    Bone marrow transplantation.
(4) X-linked.

Discussion

These investigations show that this boy has immunoglobulins present in increased concentrations and isohaemagglutinins (IgM antibodies) are present; B-cell function therefore appears normal. T-cell proliferation in response to the mitogen PHA is also unaffected and complement levels are within the reference range. However, the result of the nitroblue tetazolium (NBT) dye reduction test is diagnostic of chronic granulomatous disease (CGD). In this disorder bacteria are phagocytosed by the granulocyte, but catalase-containing bacteria cannot then be killed. The underlying abnormality is thought to be in the respiratory chain, resulting in an inability to produce superoxide radicals. When NBT is mixed with stimulated granulocytes the dye is taken up and reduced from yellow to blue (NBT-positive cells); in children with chronic granulomatous disease none of the granulocytes reacts positively. In normal children and in all other disorders of neutrophil function, apart from chronic granulomatous disease carriers, over 98% of cells will be positive if stimulated with phorbol myristate acetate (PMA). Chronic granulomatous disease is inherited, in the great majority of cases, as an X-linked disorder with female carriers showing reduced bactericidal activity.

Children with chronic granulomatous disease are susceptible to recurrent bacterial and fungal infections, particularly with *Staphylococcus aureus, Escherichia coli, Klebsiella, Serratia, Salmonella* spp., *Candida albicans, Asperillus* and *Actinomyces* spp. Treatment consists of antibiotic and antifungal chemotherapy with surgical drainage of abscesses. White cell transfusions should be given for life-threatening infections. Tissue-matched bone marrow transplantation, only possible for a few patients, offers the only hope of lasting cure.

Further reading

NELSON, pp. 519–520
SEGAL, A. W. and SOOTHILL, J. F. (1983) Defects of neutrophil function. In *Paediatric Immunology,* edited by J. F. Soothill, A. R. Hayward and C. B. S. Wood, pp. 228–247. Oxford: Blackwell Scientific Publications

Answer 49

(1) Tuberculosis.
    Leukaemia.
(2) White blood cell count.
    Culture pleural fluid – Loewenstein–Jensen media.
    Mantoux test.
    Bone marrow.

Discussion

Pleural effusions as a presentation for an underlying disease are unusual in childhood; however a knowledge of pleural fluid findings is important.

A hydrothorax develops when the plasma osmotic pressure falls and is essentially a transudate due to the negative intrapleural pressures. The fluid therefore has low specific gravity (less than 1.015), low protein content (less than 30 g/l) and contains mainly mesenchymal cells.

Purulent pleurisy leads to empyema thoracis from the adjacent infective focus which is usually obvious (pneumonia, osteomyelitis of rib, subdiaphragmatic collection, etc.. The fluid is often thick with a high specific gravity, high protein content and mainly pus cells.

Pleurisy with an effusion falls in between – the specific gravity is greater than 1.015, the protein greater than 30 g/l. Lymphocyte predominance suggests either TB or leukaemia. Mycoses are also a possibility. Neutrophil predominance would suggest a local abscess of pneumonia and the possibility of a collagen disease. Eosinophils (>10%) suggest either parasitic disease or malignancy.

Haemothorax is rare in childhood. A chylothorax may occur postoperatively or with a congenital malformation of the lymphatic system (in lymphangiectasis the fluid is milky and often contains fat globules).

Further reading

FORFAR, pp. 591, 1399
NELSON, p. 1079

Answer 50

Left ventricular hypertrophy.
ST depression with T wave inversion.

Discussion

This tracing shows a sinus tachycardia of 165 beats/min, with P waves clearly evident. The P axis and the P–R interval are both normal. The QRS axis is +100. The QRS duration is not prolonged, but left ventricular voltages are very large, with an S wave in V2 of more than 70 mm and an R wave in V6 of 32 mm. There is marked and pathological ST depression in I, II, III, V6, and AVF with accompanying biphasic T waves.

Pathological ST depression is characterized by either a downward sloping ST segment followed by inverted or biphasic T waves or an ST segment that is horizontal with a duration of more than 0.08 second. Causes of pathological ST depression with T-wave changes include, as in this case, left ventricular strain or ischaemia, digoxin, and hypokalaemia. ST depression can also occur with bundle-branch block, paroxysmal tachycardias and following ventricular extrasystoles.

ST depression is not always abnormal. In paediatric patients, non-pathological ST depression occurs in J-depression and with early repolarization. In J-depression there is a shift of the junction between the QRS and the ST segment in which case the slope of the ST segment is upwards. With early repolarization ST elevation occurs in all leads with an upright T wave and ST depression in all leads with an inverted T wave. In both J-depression and early repolarization there are no abnormal T-wave changes.

Further reading

HARRIS, L. C. and FEINSTEIN, E. (1979) *Understanding ECGs in Infants and Children*, 2nd edn. Boston: Little, Brown and Company

PARK, M. K. and GUNTHEROTH, W. G. (1981) *How to Read Pediatric ECGs*. Chicago: Year Book Medical Publishers Inc.

Answer 51

(1) Diabetic dwarfism (Maurriac's syndrome).
(2) Hypothyroidism.

Discussion

Diabetic dwarfism is due to long-standing poorly controlled diabetes mellitus and associated with hyperlipidaemia, ketosis, hyperglycaemia and hepatomegaly. Both growth and sexual development are delayed. Although this condition is rarely seen today, milder variants are not uncommon. Poor control around puberty may often be due to emotional turmoil with associated poor compliance with diet and insulin regimes.

Primary autoimmune hypothyroidism occurs more frequently in diabetics than in the general population and could also be a cause of growth and pubertal delay. However, hepatomegaly would not be a characteristic finding. Cystic fibrosis or coeliac disease can both coexist with diabetes mellitus and give stunting of growth and pubertal delay but one would expect additional symptoms.

Further reading

BAUM, J. D. (1981) Clinical management of diabetes mellitus. In *Clinical Paediatric Endocrinology*, edited by C. G. D. Brook, pp. 616–636. Oxford: Blackwell Scientific Publications
NELSON, p. 1417

Answer 52

(1) Primary proximal renal tubular acidosis.
(2) Sodium bicarbonate, and potassium supplements.

Discussion

Metabolic acidosis combined with hyperchloraemia and a normal anion gap is due to renal tubular acidosis (RTA). This boy has a normal creatinine excluding any significant reduction in glomerular filtration rate. The urine is appropriately acidic (pH<5.5); he therefore has a proximal renal tubular acidosis. There is no glycosuria or aminoaciduria as seen in secondary proximal renal tubular acidosis (Fanconi's syndrome) and so the diagnosis is primary proximal renal tubular acidosis.

Primary proximal renal tubular acidosis occurs more commonly in boys. Presentation is usually within the first 18 months and consists of persistent vomiting and growth failure. As with Fanconi's syndrome, there is a defect in proximal tubular reabsorption of bicarbonate. This is lost in the urine until plasma levels of bicarbonate are significantly reduced, at which point urinary loss ceases and an acidic urine can be generated.

Bicarbonate is given in order to maintain a normal plasma level; up to 15 mmol/kg per 24 h may be required. Potassium loss is excessive, and supplementation is necessary. In acutely ill children oral therapy is likely to be inadequate.

Further reading

MORRIS, R. C. and SEBASTIAN, A. (1983) Renal tubular acidosis and the Fanconi syndrome. In *The Metabolic Basis of Inherited Diseases,* edited by J. B. Stanbury, J. B. Wyngaarden, D. S. Fredrickson, J. L. Goldstein and M. S. Brown, pp. 1803–1843. New York: McGraw-Hill Book Company
NELSON, pp. 1344–1347

Answer 53

(1) 46XYt(21,14).
(2) Ten per cent.

Discussion

The mother is phenotypically normal having a balanced translocation between her 21 and 14 chromosomes.

Her son inherits the 'double' chromosome 14 (with the 21 attached). His total number of chromosomes is 46, he is male (46XY) and has a translocated 21 on his 14 chromosomes (46XYt(21,14)).

The risks to conceptuses can be seen from the following diagram:

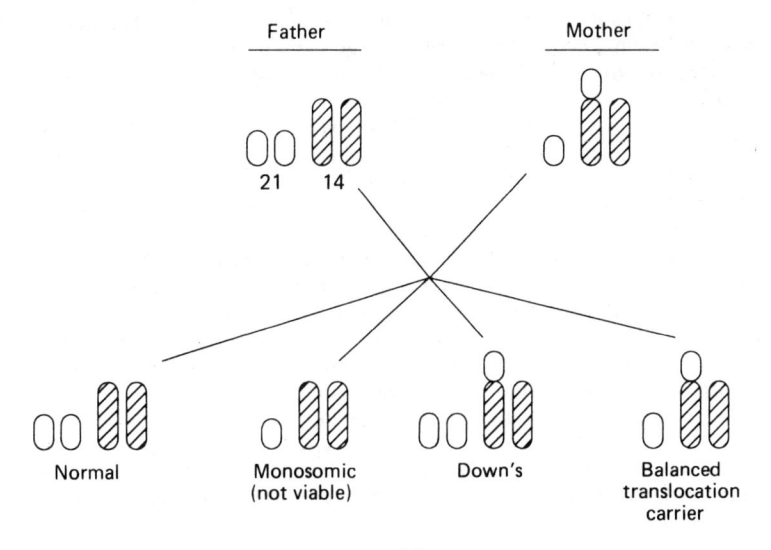

i.e. a 1:4 chance of being Down's and a 1:4 of being monosomic for chromosome 21. Monosomy-21 is non-viable and so the chances of Down's syndrome are 1 in 3 but in fact the majority of Down's syndrome fetuses are aborted and the risk decreases to about 1:10 (10%).

Interestingly, had the father been the carrier the risk would be lower still (about 2.5%) as the translocated sperms are less mobile and so less likely to form a conceptus.

Answer 54

(1) α_1-Antitrypsin deficiency.
(2) Emphysema.

Discussion

Prolonged neonatal jaundice can be due to a number of disorders and one should know at least the commoner causes. These include breast milk jaundice, neonatal hepatitis, biliary atresia, congenital infections, hypothyroidism and various metabolic disorders such as galactosaemia and α_1-antitrypsin deficiency. It is important to exclude biliary obstruction which may be surgically correctable. Here the isotope liver scan shows isotope excreted into the small bowel indicating patency of the biliary tree. This infant has an α_1-antitrypsin phenotype of PiZZ and the hepatitis is therefore most likely to be due to α_1-antitrypsin deficiency.

α_1-Antitrypsin deficiency is a genetic defect of glycoprotein metabolism and the commonest metabolic disorder associated with liver disease in infants. In those with this condition there is an absent or reduced α_1-globulin peak on serum electrophoresis. If this is found to be the case then α_1-antitrypsin levels should be measured and Pi phenotyping undertaken.

α_1-Antitrypsin is a protease inhibitor (Pi). The phenotype is inherited as an autosomal co-dominant with a large degree of genetic polymorphism. Phenotypes are designated by letters according to the electrophoretic mobility of the protein: PiM (medium fast), PiS (slow) and PiZ (ultra-slow). The level of α_1-antitrypsin varies with the phenotype. In PiMM, the commonest phenotype, this level is normal, whereas deficiency states are associated with PiZZ, PiSZ, PiZ-, and Pi- (Pi null), the percentage activity of PiMM values being 15, 35, 8, and 0, respectively.

Up to 20% of neonates with the PiZZ α_1-antitrypsin deficiency phenotype develop neonatal giant cell hepatitis in the first 4 weeks of life. One-third of these go on to develop fatal liver cirrhosis. α_1-Antitrypsin is synthesized in hepatocytes, but there is a defect in the final glycosylation, leading to a failure of secretion. It is thought likely that liver damage is associated with a viral infection or some other trigger factor.

Liver biopsy initially shows a giant cell hepatitis, and it is usually only after 3 months that globules of α_1-antitrypsin can be seen within the cytoplasm of the cell. This characteristic feature becomes present in all those with the PiZZ phenotype even if they do not have clinical evidence of liver disease.

α_1-Antitrypsin deficiency is often not associated with symptomatic disease, but a proportion of individuals will develop lower lobe emphysema in early adult life and there is also a very rare association with membranoproliferative glomerulonephritis.

Further reading

TARLOW, M. J. (1984) Liver disorders in chemical pathology. In *Chemical Pathology in the Sick Child*, edited by B. E. Clayton and J. M. Round, pp. 176–212. Oxford: Blackwell Scientific Publications

WALKER-SMITH, J. A., HAMILTON, J. R. and WALKER, W. A. (1983) Disorders of the liver – primary and secondary. In *Practical Paediatric Gastroenterology*, pp. 333–378. London: Butterworths

Answer 55

(1) Sickle-cell β^0-thalassaemia.
(2) One parent will have HbS and HbA present (sickle-cell trait), the other will have a raised level of HbF and HbA$_2$ (thalassaemia minor).
(3) Age of child.
   Size of spleen.
   Degree of hypersplenism.
   The number of transfusions required.

Discussion

The haemoglobin electrophoresis is consistent with sickle-cell disease; however, microcytosis (MCV <75 fl) is not found in sickle-cell homozygotes, and strongly suggests a diagnosis of sickle-cell β-thalassaemia. Furthermore, in sickle-cell disease, the spleen is usually impalpable by the age of 5 years due to repeated infarctions. The β-thalassaemia gene in this case will be β^0 as there is no HbA present. This contrasts with the β^+ gene in which there is β chain synthesis from 5 to 30% of normal. HbA$_2$ is likely to be increased. The diagnosis is confirmed by parental studies; one parent will show evidence of being heterozygote for the sickle-cell gene and the other evidence of the β-thalassaemia trait.

Patients with sickle-cell β-thalassaemia tend to be less severely affected than those with thalassaemia major or sickle-cell disease. The anaemia is usually less severe but painful crises do occur and there is significant splenomegaly. Management is as for mild sickle-cell anaemia, but, in contrast to it, hypersplenism may develop and necessitate splenectomy.

Sickle-cell haemoglobin C disease also causes splenomegaly, and haemoglobin electrophoresis may resemble that seen in sickle-cell disease although it is usually possible to identify the HbC. In such a case the blood film shows numerous target cells, and the haemoglobin averages between 9 and 10 g/dl. Painful crises may occur, although they are usually less severe, but there is a higher incidence of aseptic necrosis of the femoral head and of retinal damage. Microcytosis is not characteristic.

Further reading

FORFAR, pp. 952–956
KENDAL, A. G. (1983) Thalassaemias. *Medicine International*, **1**, 1169–1173
NELSON, pp. 1226–1229

Answer 56

(1) Hypernatraemic dehydration.
(2) Initial resuscitation with plasma or normal saline (10–20 ml/kg), then correct fluid loss and hypernatraemia slowly over 3–4 days using one-third to one-half normal saline/glucose solution with added potassium (provided urine output is satisfactory).

Discussion

Hypernatraemic dehydration (sodium >150 mmol/l) occurs when water loss exceeds that of sodium. The extracellular fluid volume is relatively well maintained but only at the expense of that of the intracellular fluid. Blood pressure may be normal or only marginally low even with large fluid losses, but neurological symptoms such as irritability and convulsions often occur. Hypocalcaemia and hypomagnesaemia are more frequently associated with this type of dehydration.

It is important that fluid replacement does not result in any rapid change in the serum sodium with an excessive osmotic fluid shift into cells. Rehydration with 5% dextrose should be avoided. Many children require initial correction of their circulating blood volume with plasma or normal saline, but subsequent treatment should aim to restore serum sodium to normal over 3–4 days, using hypotonic solutions of one-third to one-half normal saline containing adequate dextrose. Potassium supplements should be added only when there is satisfactory urine output, providing that the child is not hyperkalaemic. Metabolic acidosis will correct spontaneously with rehydration and bicarbonate is only required if it is severe.

Further reading

FORFAR, pp. 412–413
NELSON, pp. 232–238

Answer 57

(1) Normal for age!
(2) None.

Discussion

The normal range for haemoglobin at 6 months of age is 10.5–14 g/dl and, while the haemoglobin level falls just outside this range, the red blood cell indices are all within the normal range (MCV 76–88 fl, MCH 24–30 pg, MCHC 30–36 g/dl).

In an asymptomatic child no therapy is indicated.
Be careful of this type of question!!

Further reading

FORFAR, p. 1989

Answer 58

Three-and-a-half years.

Discussion

A circle is mastered about the age of 3 years; this drawing has two additional features – eyes and legs – which would score the child between 3 and 4 years on the Goodenough Draw a Man test.

Copying a ladder is a test from the Ruth Griffiths Scales of Mental Development. Horizontal and vertical strokes are clearly mastered, but there is an extra rung and the rungs do not join neatly to the verticals. An accurate (stage II) drawing can be expected by 6 years – but this drawing (stage I) would be expected at 3.5–4 years.

Answer 59

(1) Polyostotic fibrous dysplasia (McCune–Albright syndrome).
(2) Skeletal survey.
    Thyroid function tests.

Discussion

The combination of precocious puberty, cutaneous pigmentation and fibrous dysplasia is known as the McCune–Albright syndrome. Although more commonly seen in girls, it has been reported in boys.

In this child the bone age is markedly advanced, and oestradiol levels are raised (prepubertal levels <50). A skeletal survey is likely to show areas of osseous, cyst-like lesions. These bone abnormalities are in fact solid, consisting of poorly formed bone and cartilage. Children may present with pathological fractures, and deformities may result.

Other endocrine disorders, particularly hyperthyroidism and Cushing's syndrome, are not uncommon. In the former, TSH is found to be suppressed, excluding a hypothalamic cause. This raises the question as to whether the disorder is primarily one of target organ hyperactivity or initially hypothalamic in origin. All patients require full endocrine investigation.

LHRH analogues have been used to treat the precocious puberty. Hyperthyroidism and Cushing's syndrome require treatment if present. Symptomatic dysplastic bone lesions may require bone grafts. The long-term prognosis is good, although early epiphyseal fusion may occur. The bone lesions become static in adulthood.

Further reading

RAYNER, P. H. W. (1981) Early puberty. In *Clinical Paediatric Endocrinology*, edited by C. G. D. Brook, pp. 224–239 Oxford: Blackwell Scientific Publications

VISSNER, K. A. (1984) In *Chemical Pathology in the Sick Child*, edited by B. E. Clayton and J. M. Round, pp. 343–364. Oxford: Blackwell Scientific Publications

Answer 60

(1) Ventricular extrasystoles.
(2) Probably none, provided asymptomatic and extrasystoles abolished by exercise.

Discussion

This tracing shows a sinus arrhythmia with uniform ventricular extrasystoles occurring approximately once every 3 seconds.

Ventricular extrasystoles (also termed 'ventricular premature beats') are characterized by wide abnormal looking QRS complexes unrelated to the P wave. The electrical impulse from the extrasystole is usually blocked by the AV node (this depends, among other factors, on the degree of prematurity). The SA node is therefore not depolarized by retrograde conduction, its rate remains unaffected and there is a full compensatory pause following each SA node impulse. The time between two normal QRS complexes will thus be half that between two QRS complexes that are interrupted by a ventricular extrasystole. Extrasystoles usually arise from a single ventricular focus if they are of identical configuration in the same lead, but may arise from separate foci if their configuration changes (hence termed 'multiform').

Ventricular bigeminy (coupling) occurs if each ventricular extrasystole alternates regularly with a normal ventricular complex.

In children, ventricular asystoles are usually benign if they are infrequent, uniform, and abolished by exercise. In such cases treatment is not normally required. However, those that are either associated with severe heart disease, occur frequently, are multiform, induced by exercise, or coupled (ventricular bigeminy) are usually significant.

Ventricular extrasystoles may also be secondary to hypoxia, electrolyte disturbances, drugs including digoxin (which characteristically causes bigeminy), quinine and tricyclics, and myocarditis.

Further reading

HARRIS, L. C. and FEINSTEIN, E. (1979) *Understanding ECGs in Infants and Children*, 2nd edn. Boston: Little, Brown and Company
JORDON, S. C. and AND SCOTT, O. (1981) *Heart Disease in Paediatrics*, 2nd edn, pp. 304–306 London: Butterworths
PARK, M. K. and GUNTHEROTH, W. G. (1981) *How to Read Pediatric ECGs*. Chicago: Year Book Medical Publishers Inc

Answer 61

(1) Turner's syndrome.
(2) Lymphocytic thyroiditis (Hashimoto's disease).
(3) Antithyroid antibodies.

Discussion

Children with Turner's syndrome have an increased incidence of lymphocytic thyroiditis, although the reason for this association is unknown. In lymphocytic thyroiditis, thyroid function may be normal but TSH is often raised, as in this girl. A T_4 of 70 nmol/l is within the normal range; hypothyroidism is unlikely to have made any significant contribution to her short stature. Antithyroglobulin antibodies by radio-immunoassay are found in >90% of cases of lymphocytic thyroiditis, whereas microsomal antithyroid antibodies are found in 60%. Antithyroid antibodies are also present in an increased percentage of mothers of children with Turner's syndrome. Children with Noonan's and Down's syndrome also have a higher incidence of this disorder.

Further reading

MALVAUX, P. (1981) Hypothyroidism. In *Clinical Paediatric Endocrinology*, edited by C. G. D. Brook, pp. 329–339. Oxford: Blackwell Scientific Publications
NELSON, pp. 1461–1462; p. 1501

Answer 62

(1) Compensated respiratory acidosis.
(2) Cystic fibrosis.

Discussion

The pH is in the normal range and therefore the child is not acidotic. However, the $P\text{co}_2$ is high as is the bicarbonate, suggesting either a compensated respiratory acidosis or, conversely, a compensated metabolic alkalosis; as a respiratory disorder is suggested by the nasal polyps and the low $P\text{o}_2$, the former interpretation is correct.

Nasal polyposis is a well recognized complication of cystic fibrosis and, while it is an unusual presentation, milder variants of cystic fibrosis are increasingly being recognized.

Further reading

FLAKE, C. G., KULCZYCKI, L. L., MUELLER, H. L. and SHWACHMAN, H. (1962) Nasal polyposis in patients with cystic fibrosis. *Pediatrics*, **30**, 387

Answer 63

(1) Rotor syndrome.
(2) Bromsulphthalein excretion test; urinary coproporphyrins.
    Oral cholecystogram.

Discussion

Dubin–Johnson and Rotor syndrome are both rare inherited syndromes of conjugated hyperbilirubinaemia with little in the way of signs and symptoms other than jaundice.

Dubin–Johnson syndrome usually presents after puberty – the jaundice increasing with intercurrent infection, oral contraceptives and pregnancy.

Rotor syndrome presents at a younger age, the prognosis being good – the condition persists but does not progress.

The investigations presented show a mild elevation of liver enzymes. The bile in the urine shows a conjugated hyperbilirubinaemia.

Investigative results can be summarized as follows:

	Rotor	*Dubin–Johnson*
Urinary coproporphyrins	Total raised <80% coproporphyrin 1	Total normal >80% coproporphyrin 1
BSP at 45 min	Elevated No 90 min secondary rise	Normal 90 min secondary rise demonstrated
Oral cholecystogram	Gallbladder seen	Gallbladder not seen
Liver biopsy	Normal	Interlobular pigmentation of hepatocytes with lipofuscin staining

Further reading

FORFAR, p. 1240
STANBURY, J. B. (1983) *The Metabolic Basis of Inherited Disease*, 5th edn., p. 1408. New York: McGraw-Hill

Answer 64

(1) Bilateral high frequency hearing loss.
(2) Genetic.
   Rubella.
   Postmeningitis.

Discussion

The prevalence in the general population of sensorineural deafness is about 1 in 1000. There is a male predominance and there is a slight increase in lower social classes.

The largest group is of unknown aetiology, but where a cause is known the order in decreasing frequency is as follows: (1) genetic (about half are autosomal dominant and half autosomal recessive); (2) perinatal, i.e. hypoxia, infection, jaundice; (3) rubella associated, and (4) postnatal, e.g. trauma, meningitis, cardiac arrest, post-surgery, and then miscellaneous causes including congenital malformations, cytomegalovirus.

Answer 65

(1) Idiopathic hypercalcaemia.
(2) Correct dehydration and induce diuresis with frusemide.
    Low calcium and low vitamin D diet.
    Prednisolone in refractory cases.

Discussion

This girl has a very high serum calcium, with a normal phosphate and low alkaline phosphatase. These findings together with the clinical details as given are most likely to be due to idiopathic hypercalcaemia. This is a condition of unknown aetiology, thought to be due to an abnormal sensitivity to vitamin D. It is now rare, although the incidence was higher when fortified milks were used.

Idiopathic hypercalcaemia is usually divided into mild and severe forms, although there is a degree of overlap. Children with mild disease present between 3 and 12 months of age with weight loss, vomiting, constipation and irritability. Those with 'severe' disease are of low birth weight, have a characteristic facies (low set ears, squint, hypertelorism, prominent cheeks, and an upturned nose with a flattened nasal bridge), and are developmentally delayed. On examination they usually have a raised blood pressure and a systolic murmur (due to supravalvular aortic stenosis and/or pulmonary artery stenosis).

With treatment, full recovery is usual in those with the mild disease, but if untreated permanent renal, cerebral and cardiac damage can occur. Death may follow renal failure or intercurrent infection. In severe cases the degree to which treatment affects the outcome is less clear. Very high serum calcium levels can be reduced within a few hours by inducing diuresis with frusemide; intravenous fluids with added sodium supplementation are usually required to avoid dehydration and hyponatraemia. Vitamin D should be excluded from the diet, a low calcium milk formula used (e.g. Locasol) and prednisolone started in those cases refractory to dietary changes alone. Attention should also be paid to the calcium content of the local water supply; distilled water is used to reconstitute Locasol.

Vitamin D in gross overdosage (hypervitaminosis D) can also cause hypercalcaemia, a low alkaline phosphatase and a variable phosphate level.

Further reading

AARSKOG, D. (1981) Dysmorphic syndromes. In *Clinical Paediatric Endocrinology*, edited by C. G. D. Brook, pp. 159–190. Oxford: Blackwell Scientific Publications

GERTNER, J. M. (1984) Disorders of bone and mineral metabolism. In *Chemical Pathology in the Sick Child*, edited by B. E. Clayton and J. M. Round, pp. 365–404. Oxford: Blackwell Scientific Publications

Answer 66

Iron deficiency.
β-Thalassaemia major or intermedia.
Haemoglobin H disease.
Chronic disease.
Lead poisoning.
Hereditary sideroblastic anaemia.
Copper deficiency.

Discussion

This is a straightforward question, assuming one knows the normal values for the red cell indices, and asking the causes of a microcytic, hypochromic anaemia. In this boy both the MCV and the MCHC are low (normal range: MCV 76–96 fl; MCHC 32–36 g/dl).

Iron deficiency is confirmed either by a low serum iron combined with an increase in total iron-binding capacity (TIBC), or by the single finding of a low serum ferritin concentration. β-Thalassaemia major or intermedia could be associated with a haemoglobin of this level, but in thalassaemia minor anaemia is usually mild. HbH disease, an α-thalassaemia in which there is deletion of three of the four genes coding for the α-chain, can cause a moderately severe haemolytic anaemia with microcytosis. α-Thalassaemia 1, where two of the four α-chain genes are deleted, also causes microcytosis but only a mild anaemia. In thalassaemia both the serum iron and serum ferritin are raised, while the TIBC is normal. Hb electrophoresis and HbA_2 and HbF quantification are required to establish the diagnosis.

The anaemia of chronic disease, for example, in chronic juvenile arthritis, is usually a mild normochromic anaemia but may be hypochromic and occasionally also microcytic. The serum iron is reduced but ferritin levels are high. The TIBC is usually normal.

Chronic lead poisoning causes anaemia by interfering with iron utilization and haem synthesis. Red cells have a characteristic basophilic stippling, free erythrocyte porphyrin and the urinary excretion of coproporphyrins and δ-aminolaevulinic acid is raised. Blood lead will be greater than 1.4 μmol/l.

Hereditary sideroblastic anaemia, an inherited sex-linked recessive condition, is characterized by a hypochromic microcytic anaemia. The bone marrow contains nucleated red cells with haemosiderin granules surrounding the nuclei (ringed sideroblasts). Serum iron levels are raised. A number of these children respond to treatment with pyridoxine (vitamin B_6).

Copper deficiency can cause a hypochromic anaemia refractory to iron therapy but it is usually accompanied by neutropenia.

Further reading

FITZSIMONS, E. and JACOBS, A. (1983) Iron deficiency anaemia. *Medicine International*, **1**, 1155
KENDALL, A. G. (1983) Thalassaemias. *Medicine International*, **1**, 1169–1173
NELSON, pp. 1214–1217

Answer 67

(1) Trisomy-18 – Edward's syndrome.
(2) Overlapping – index and middle fingers – a flexion deformity.
    Hypoplasia of the little fingernails.
    Simple arch dermatoglyphics.

Discussion

It is important to be able to decipher photographs of chromosomes (karyotypes). The layout of the chromosomes is by size and centromere position – starting in the top left with the large chromosomes with the median centromeres. Progressing to the right within the group of like-sized chromosomes, the centromere moves distally to produce submetacentric and acrocentric chromosomes. Chromosomes therefore fall naturally into seven groups (A–G). This is known as the Patau classification.

This child has a trisomy of one of the small chromosomes with median/submetacentric centromeres – an E-group trisomy – in this particular case trisomy-18. The exact chromosome within the group is decided by banding techniques.

Further reading

FORFAR, p. 910

Answer 68

(1) Hereditary angioneurotic oedema.
(2) Androgens (danazol).
    ε-Aminocaproic acid.
    Tranexamic acid.
(3) Respiratory obstruction due to laryngeal oedema.

Discussion

Hereditary angioneurotic oedema is a disorder caused by deficiency of the enzyme C1 esterase inhibitor (C1 INH), the only known inhibitor of activated C1s. Inheritance is autosomal dominant. Clinical manifestations include non-itchy localized skin swellings lasting several days (in contrast to allergic urticaria), colicky abdominal pain and, more seriously, laryngeal oedema. Serum concentrations of C1 esterase inhibitor are less than one-third of normal, and fall to very low levels during attacks. Uninhibited activation of C1 results in excessive cleavage of C2 and C4, with a subsequent reduction in the serum concentrations, although these are normal between attacks. C2b, a product of C2 cleavage, is split by plasmin to produce a vasoactive fragment. In approximately 15% of patients, C1 esterase inhibitor levels as measured by immunoassay are normal but the enzyme is non-functional. It is, therefore, essential to use a functional assay in patients with clinical symptoms of this disease, even if C1 esterase inhibitor levels, measured by immunoassay, are within the reference range.

Treatment with a low dose androgen such as danazol is an effective prophylactic agent, inducing synthesis of C1 esterase inhibitor or, in those with non-functioning enzyme, both suppressing synthesis of the abnormal non-functioning protein and stimulating production of the normal enzyme. ε-Aminocaproic acid, tranexamic acid or fresh frozen plasma have also been used in treatment.

Further reading

ATHERTON, D. J. (1983) Immunological aspects of skin diseases. In *Paediatric Immunology*, edited by J. F. Soothill, A. R. Hayward and C. B. S. Wood, pp. 393–426. Oxford: Blackwell Scientific Publications
NELSON, p. 515
TURNER, M. W. (1983) Complement defects. In *Paediatric Immunology*, edited by J. F. Soothill, A. R. Hayward and C. B. S. Wood, pp. 212–227. Oxford: Blackwell Scientific Publications

Answer 69

(1) Haemoglobinuria.
(2) Yes – haemolysis.
(3) Red cell glucose-6-phosphate dehydrogenase activity.

Discussion

Questions with a haematological bias and involving Filipinos, Thais, Chinese, Greeks, Italians and Africans should alert you to the possibility of glucose-6-phosphate dehydrogenase deficiency.

There are two clinical syndromes involved: the first is haemolysis related to ingestion of drugs, fava beans or intercurrent infection. The second is a chronic non-spherocytic haemolytic anaemia.

The question describes the former syndrome resulting in haemoglobinuria once plasma haptoglobulins are saturated.

Whether sulphasalazine should be discontinued depends on the severity of the underlying disease compared to the severity of the anaemia. Eventually the patient will compensate by having a faster red cell turnover.

Other drugs which may lead to haemolysis include phenacetin, aspirin, sulphonamides, vitamin K, primaquine, chloramphenicol, nitrofurantoin. The ingestion of fava beans may also provoke episodes of haemolysis in affected subjects.

Further reading

FORFAR, pp. 950, 1233
NELSON, p. 1222

Answer 70

(1) Atrial flutter.
(2) Digoxin.
    DC cardioversion.

Discussion

Atrial flutter can be recognized by the characteristic 'saw tooth' F or flutter waves (with a rate of 300–400 impulses/min). The AV node is unable to respond to the rapid atrial frequency and there is subsequently a degree of AV block. The ventricular rate will be regular if this is fixed (at 2:1, 3:1 or 4:1 etc.), but irregular if it varies.

In this ECG the atrial rate is approximately 375/min. Although the AV conduction may appear irregular this is actually 2:1 block high in the AV node and 3:2 Wenckebach conduction lower in the AV node. The QRS complex thus occurs in pairs. The average ventricular rate is approximately 130/min.

Atrial flutter is rare in children but it can occur following cardiac surgery involving the atria (e.g. for ostium secundum atrial septal defect, total anomalous pulmonary venous drainge, and transposition), in structual defects with atrial dilatation, in myocarditis and with acute infections. It may alternate with atrial fibrillation. Atrial flutter can also be an isolated neonatal arrhythmia, with a low recurrence risk and an excellent prognosis.

Digoxin remains the drug of choice for atrial flutter. By increasing the AV block it slows the ventricular rate and may spontaneously convert flutter to either atrial fibrillation or sinus rhythm. Disopyramide is also used in digitalized patients with atrial flutter. Cardioversion is the treatment of choice in children who are critically ill or who have a 1:1 AV conduction with a very rapid ventricular rate. It is also very successful in converting flutter to sinus rhythm in children with underlying heart disease. Intractable atrial flutter should be treated with digoxin with the addition of verapamil or a β-blocker if necessary.

Further reading

PARK, M. C. and GUNTHEROTH, W. G. (1981) *How to Read Pediatric ECGs*. Chicago: Year Book Medical Publishers Inc.

Answer 71

(1) 'Central' diabetes insipidus.
(2) Optic atrophy.
(3) DIDMOAD syndrome (Wolfram syndrome).

Discussion

In the water deprivation test a urine osmolality of less than 100 mosmol/kg with a plasma osmolality of >305 mosmol/kg, after a weight loss of 5%, is usually indicative of central (hypothalamic) diabetes insipidus (DI). This is confirmed by an increase in urine osmolality of >50% following the administration of desmopressin. In a normal individual urine osmalitity will rise spontaneously to >850 mosmol/kg, whereas in renal diabetes insipidus there will be no significant increase in osmality with exogenous desmopressin.

The DIDMOAD syndrome (diabetes insipidus, diabetes mellitus, optic atrophy and deafness) or Wolfram syndrome is a rare autosomal recessive disorder. Diabetes mellitus usually presents in the first decade and in approximately one-third of affected children is followed in the second decade by diabetes insipidus, although the appearance of different components of the syndrome may vary. Optic atrophy is progressive and may lead to blindness in adulthood, whereas the bilateral high tone deafness is not usually of clinical significance.

Further reading

NELSON, pp. 1437–1440
PERHEENTUPA, J. (1981) The neurohypophysis and water regulation. In *Clinical Paediatric Endocrinology*, edited by C. G. D. Brook, pp. 305–325. Oxford: Blackwell Scientific Publications

Answer 72

(1) Fanconi's syndrome.
(2) Cystinosis.
    Galactosaemia.
    Wilson's disease.
    Hereditary fructose intolerance.
    Lowe's occulocerebral degeneration.
    Tyrosinosis.
    Heavy metals.
    Outdated tetracyclines.

Discussion

A low plasma phosphate, a low normal plasma calcium and a raised alkaline phosphatase are all findings compatible with rickets. Aminoaciduria and a decreased percentage tubular reabsorption of phosphate (%TPR) (normal >80%) are not exclusive to Fanconi's syndrome and may be found in some other causes of rickets. However, this child has a renal tubular acidosis, as evidenced by hyperchloraemic acidosis, with a normal anion gap and hypokalaemia. Proximal renal tubular acidosis with generalized aminoaciduria and glycosuria are the main features of this syndrome.

There are a number of disorders in which Fanconi's syndrome is found, including an idiopathic 'adult' variety. In this child, the most likely cause is cystinosis which should be confirmed by looking for an increased level of cystine in leucocytes and cystine crystals in the cornea on slit light examination. Cystine crystals are also found in the rectal mucosa, bone marrow and lymph nodes. Do not confuse cystinosis with cystinuria, which is neither associated with extrarenal cystine deposition nor with Fanconi's syndrome. Other causes are listed above.

Further reading

FORFAR, p. 1227–1228
MORRIS, R. C. and SEBASTIAN, A. (1983) Renal tubular acidosis and the Fanconi syndrome. In *The Metabolic Basis of Inherited Diseases*, edited by J. B. Stanbury, J. B. Wyngaarden, D. S. Fredrickson, J. L. Goldstein and M. S. Brown, pp. 1803–1843. New York: McGraw-Hill Book Company
NELSON, pp. 1660–1661, 1344–1347
SCHNEIDER, J. A. and SCHULMAN, J. D. (1983) Cystinosis. In *The Metabolic Basis of Inherited Diseases*, edited by J. B. Stanbury, J. B. Wyngaarden, D. S. Fredrickson, J. L. Goldstein and M. S. Brown, pp. 1844–1866. New York: McGraw–Hill Book Company

Answer 73

(1) Restrictive lung function and hypoventilation.
(2) EMG.
    Tensilon (edrophonium chloride) test.
(3) Juvenile myasthenia gravis.

Discussion

Both the FEV_1 and the FVC are reduced proportionately – hence the normal FEV_1/FVC ratio.

The child is hypoventilating – shown by the raised Pco_2 and low Po_2 with a lowish pH suggesting an acute or chronic respiratory acidosis.

Myasthenia gravis is often subtle in its initial presentation. The symptoms are often vague but fatiguability (or improvement after resting) is a feature which may not always be enquired after.

Ptosis is the most common presentation, but ophthamoplegia and facial weakness commonly occur. It is about six times more common in girls than boys and the incidence ranges from 0.5 to 3 per 1000 of which 1% are children.

EMG would show polyphasic action potentials of short duration suggestive of a myopathy. The Tensilon test is diagnostic – the improvement is almost instantaneous and lasts about 5 minutes.

Further reading

FORFAR, p. 847
NELSON, p. 1607
SWAINMAN K. F. and WRIGHT F. S. (1982) *The Practice of Pediatric Neurology*, 2nd edn., p. 1207. New York: C. V. Mosby

Answer 74

Infection.
Glucose-6-phosphate dehydrogenase deficiency.
HbH disease.
Severe bruising.
Hereditary spherocytosis.
Hereditary elliptocytosis.
Pyruvate kinase deficiency.

Discussion

Haemolysis is the most likely cause of jaundice in a neonate who is anaemic. Physiological jaundice is not associated with anaemia, neither should it present in the first 24 hours nor be so severe. Haemolysis can be divided into two groups on the basis of the direct Coombs' test (DCT).

A positive direct Coombs' test is seen in rhesus disease although it may only be weakly positive in ABO incompatibility. Other blood group incompatibilities (e.g. Duffy, Kell and Kidd) causing this degree of haemolysis should give a positive Coombs' test.

Haemolytic anaemia with a negative direct Coombs' test could be due to congenital or acquired infections, disorders of red cell morphology (hereditary spherocytosis and hereditary elliptocytosis), deficiencies of the red cell enzymes, glucose-6-phosphate dehydrogenase or pyruvate kinase, or α-thalassaemia.

Glucose-6-phosphate dehydrogenase deficiency is common in black, Oriental and Mediterranean people, but is most severe in the latter two groups. Inheritance is sex-linked recessive. Oxidative haemolysis can occur in the absence of oxidant drugs and may be precipitated by infection.

Pyruvate kinase deficiency leads to a decrease in red cell ATP, potassium leak from the cell, and its lifespan is significantly reduced. Inheritance is autosomal recessive. Hexokinase deficiency and galactosaemia may also be associated with haemolysis in the neonatal period.

α-Thalassaemia is common in Chinese and, unlike β-thalassaemia, can present in the newborn since HbF contains α-chains. In HbH disease there are deletions on chromosome 16 of three of the four genes which code for the α-chain. On haemoglobin electrophoresis at birth up to 25% of haemoglobin is HbBarts (4 γ-chains) but this is soon replaced by HbH (4 β-chains).

Extravascular haemolysis from birth trauma (e.g. cephalhaematoma or other bruising) may be severe enough to result in a fall in haemoglobin and subsequent jaundice.

Further reading

FORFAR, pp. 197–199
NELSON, pp. 383–388

POLAND, L. and OSTREA, E. M. (1979) Neonatal hyperbilirubinaemia. In *Care of the High Risk Neonate*, edited by H. M. Klaus and A. A., Fanaroff, pp. 243–266. Philadelphia: W. B. Saunders

ROBERTON, N. R. C. (1986) *A Manual of Neonatal Intensive Care*. London: Edward Arnold

WILEY, J. S. (1983) The haemolytic anaemias. *Medicine International*, **1**, 1202–1206

Answer 75

(1) Rickets.
(2) Renal failure.
(3) Blood pressure.
    Haemoglobin.
    Creatinine clearance.
    Wrist X-ray.

Discussion

The biochemistry suggests the diagnosis of rickets – low calcium, high phosphorus and an alkaline phosphatase above the upper limit of normal for age. An X-ray of the wrist would confirm this.

The underlying diagnosis of chronic renal failure is evident by the high creatinine and potassium.

Important immediate investigations are his haemoglobin (it is suggested he is pale), his blood pressure (not mentioned) and creatinine clearance. The results of each would influence acute management.

In the longer term the cause of his renal failure would need to be established – investigation might include intravenous urogram (IVU), micturating cystogram, DMSA (2,3-dimercaptosuccinic acid) and DTPA (diethyltriamine pentaacetic acid) isotope scans.

Further reading

FORFAR, p. 1299

Answer 76

(1) Yes.
(2) −170 daPa.
(3) A blocked eustachian tube.

Discussion

Tympanometry is the measuremennt of the mobility of the tympanic membrane: conditions such as perforation, blocked eustachian tubes and serous otitis media will be revealed.

Tympanometry is one facet of the examination of the audiological system and cannot be taken in isolation from history, examination and audiological assessment.

The tympanic membrane is most able to vibrate (i.e. most compliant) when the pressures on either side are equal. The tympanogram probe is a tight fit in the external auditory canal. The machine generates negative and positive pressures (horizontal axis), while measuring the sound level in the external auditory canal produced by a small loudspeaker in the probe.

The sound level measured is at its lowest when the sound is transmitted by the tympanic membrane. This is inverted to form the vertical axis.

In the normal ear the 'peak' is at 0 pressure because the middle ear is aerated via the eustachian tube.

In this case the eustachian tube is blocked, oxygen has been absorbed from the trapped air in the middle ear, so creating a negative pressure in the middle ear. The result is that the tympanic membrane is most compliant at $-170\,\text{daPa}$.

As the tympanic membrane has retained its normal mobility, albeit at a negative pressure, hearing is not affected.

Below is a normal tympanogram (solid line), a hypermobile drum (dashed line) and a stiff drum (dotted line).

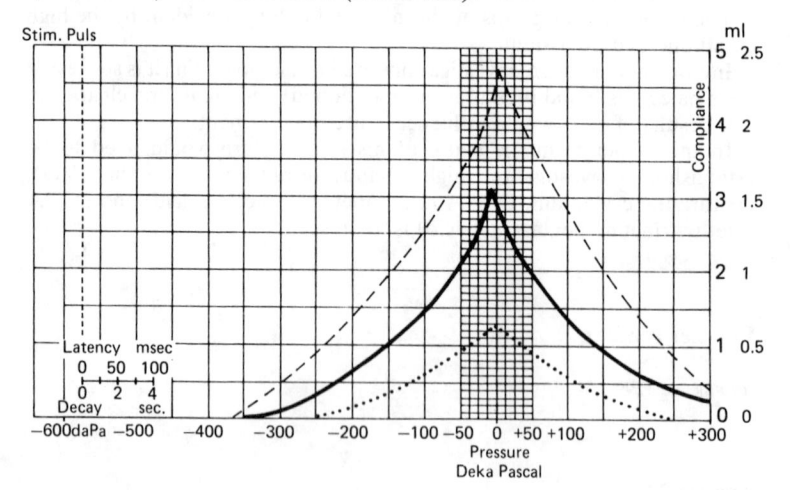

Further reading

FORFAR, p. 750

Answer 77

The child's age is 4.5–5 years.

Discussion

This may seem to be an unfair question as it gives insufficient information about the quality of the drawing. You have to presume that they are copied accurately.

For your information the following may be helpful estimations – all are copied shapes.

Scribble	18–28 months
Circular scribble	2.5–3 years
Horizontal line	3 years
Vertical line	3 years
Circle	3 years
Cross	4 years
Square	5 years
Triangle	6 years
Diamond	7 years

All these figures are approximate and most children will achieve the items by the ages stated.

Answer 78

(1) Respiratory alkalosis.
(2) Hysteria.

Discussion

Information is often omitted from data interpretation questions in order to concentrate on the data.

In this question you would like to know that a detailed history, physical examination and probably chest X-ray are normal before concluding this is hysterical.

Having said that, it is unusual to produce a respiratory alkalosis (with a normal Po_2 breathing room air) and so it must be concluded that there is an element of anxiety or hysteria present.

Overdose of a respiratory stimulant, raised intracranial pressure, or brainstem lesion or the very early stages of salicylate overdose should be considered, but would not usually present with chest pain.

Some 'organic' presentations of hysteria can be very difficult to correctly diagnose – sometimes the child can be 'tricked' into revealing inconsistencies on examination. Sometimes a short period of observation in hospital is preferable to extensive investigation.

When hysteria is diagnosed it is important to look into precipitating causes and provide appropriate help.

Further reading

FORFAR, p. 1805
NELSON, p. 1554

Answer 79

(1) 1:2.
(2) None but 1:2 will be carriers.

Discussion

All forms of glucose-6-phosphate dehydrogenase deficiency are inherited as a sex-linked character with intermediate dominance. Males who are hemizygous are therefore always affected but heterozygous females will be affected to a minor degree. They have two distinct populations of red cells – one deficient the other not deficient – an example of the Lyon hypothesis of random X-chromosome inactivation.

Male offspring will have a 1:2 chance of being affected. Female offspring will not be affected but 1:2 will be carriers and will have reduced enzyme levels on testing.

Answer 80

(1) Third degree heart block.
(2) Congenital.
(3) None.

Discussion

On this tracing, the atrial rate is approximately 80/min and the ventricular rate 42/min. Both are regular. QRS complexes appear normal. Ventricular depolarization is entirely independent of that of the atria and this is therefore an example of complete (third degree) heart block.

Complete heart block (CHB) may be either congenital or acquired. In the congenital form the pacemaker is usually above the bifurcation of the bundle of His in the AV node. QRS complexes are of normal appearance and the ventricular rate often slows with rest and increases with exercise. Congenital heart block can occur with structural defects (e.g. congenitally corrected transposition of the great arteries), but in the majority of cases the heart is otherwise normal. In 30% of cases of neonatal congenital complete heart block there is a maternal connective tissue disease. Treatment is only required if symptoms are present (syncope or congestive failure) or if 24-hour ECG monitoring shows dangerously slow rates.

In acquired lesions the pacemaker is in most cases below the bifurcation of the bundle of His. The QRS complexes resemble ventricular premature beats. Acquired lesions may be a result of cardiac surgery (there is a 1–2% incidence following ventricular septal defect closure), myocarditis (e.g. rheumatic fever or diphtheria) or following myocardial infarction (very rare in children). Acquired lesions should be treated with pacing.

Further reading

PARK, M. K. and GUNTHEROTH, W. G. (1981) *How to Read Pediatric ECGs.* Chicago: Year Book Medical Publishers Inc.

Answer 81

(1) Somogyi effect.
(2) Gradual reduction in insulin dosage.

Discussion

Most pre-adolescent children with diabetes require less than 1 unit of insulin per kg per 24 hours to maintain good control. In those where control is inadequate, but are on a dose greater than this, it is important to exclude the Somogyi effect. The Somogyi effect consists of nocturnal hypoglycaemia with a rebound release of insulin antagonists causing hyperglycaemia, hyperlipidaemia, and ketonaemia. The nocturnal hypoglycaemia may or may not be apparent; children may have nightmares or wake up. The first morning urine specimen may contain ketones only, or ketones and glucose, depending on the time of voiding in relationship to that of the hypoglycaemia. The diagnosis is confirmed by documenting the nocturnal hypoglycaemia and treatment consists of grandually reducing the total dose of insulin or, if this is not excessive, in reducing the insulin that is active at the time the hypoglycaemia occurs.

Other explanations for nocturnal hypoglycaemia with poor day time control, based upon variations in insulin absorptions, have also been suggested.

Further reading

BELTON, N. R. and FARQUHAR, J. W. (1984) Diabetes mellitus. In *Chemical Pathology in the Sick Child,* edited by B. E. Clayton and J. M. Round, pp. 265-295. Oxford: Blackwell Scientific Publications
FORFAR, p. 1184
NELSON, p. 1415

Answer 82

(1) Autoimmune haemolytic anaemia.
(2) White cell count, platelet count.

Discussion

This child is anaemic and mildly jaundiced and the reticulocyte count is raised. The positive Coombs' test indicates the presence of antibodies to red blood cells.

The exact aetiology of acquired haemolytic anaemias is unknown but they fall into three groups:

(1) Acute transient early childhood – usually following an infection (often respiratory) that is followed by 'acute' haemolysis leading to pallor, jaundice, splenomegaly and haemoglobinuria. It responds to steroids and usually resolves within 3 months.
(2) Chronic later childhood – there may be some underlying cause, e.g. drugs, reticulosis, systemic lupus erythematosus etc. Abnormalities of other blood elements often coexist. The response to steroids is variable and a relapsing course is not unusual. The mortality may be as high as 10% depending upon the underlying condition.

Both these forms of autoimmune haemolytic anaemia involve mainly IgG with complement activation – this occurs maximally at 37°C and so these are called 'warm antibodies'.

(3) Autoimmune haemolytic anaemia associated with 'cold' antibodies usually occurs following viral infections (e.g. infectious mononucleosis) and mycoplasma pneumonia and the haemolysis may be triggered by exposure to cold. The antibody responsible is of the IgM type. The prognosis is usually good.

Further reading
FORFAR, p. 956
NELSON, p. 1229
SOOTHILL, J. F. (1983) In *Paediatric Immunology*, edited by J. F. Soothill, A. R. Hayward and C. B. S. Wood. Oxford: Blackwell Scientific

Answer 83

(1) Enzyme induction or inadequate dosage.
(2) Enzyme induction or inadequate dosage.
(3) Anticonvulsant-induced rickets.
(4) Anticonvulsant-induced rickets.
(5) Rickets or normal growth.
(6) Post-convulsion.

Discussion

This question usually appears with three of the branches revolving around either enzyme induction leading to increased metabolism of the anticonvulsants themselves or of vitamin D and subsequent rickets. Where the calcium and phosphorus values are normal, then the explanation for the alkaline phosphatase being outside the normal adult range is normal childhood growth. The high creatinine kinase value merely reflects continuous strenuous muscular activity secondary to the convulsion.

Inadequate dosage or inadequate compliance is often the cause of poor seizure control – this child's phenytoin levels are normal so it is presumed that the child is receiving treatment as prescribed.

Answer 84

(1) Galactosaemia; rubella infection.
(2) Urine reducing substances and, if positive, red cell galactose-1-phosphate uridyl transferase assay.
   TORCH screen.
   Septic screen.
(3) Stop feeds.
   Intravenous fluids and antibiotics.
   Monitor jaundice.
   Check maternal rubella status.

Discussion

The key to this question is the red reflexes which are poorly seen, coupled with an enlarged liver and jaundice.

Rubella produces corneal clouding, while galactosaemia produces lens opacities; both produce a hepatitis resulting in jaundice and failure to thrive.

It is important to act promptly in this situation as the outcome for the child with galactosaemia can be dramatically improved by the early diagnosis and a galactose-free diet. Unfortunately, the same cannot be said for the rubella baby – however careful the follow-up, looking for visual and hearing problems as well as other 'rubella complications' will help to ameliorate the condition.

In practice a septic screen should also be carried out since sepsis, although not explaining the eye abnormalities, could produce many of the symptoms described.

Answer 85

(1) Herpes simplex encephalitis.
(2) Brain biopsy.
   CT scan.
(3) Intravenous acyclovir or vidarabine.

Discussion

Herpes simplex type 1 is a common cause of sporadic encephalitis particularly in older children and adults. Neonatal infection is generalized, involves a meningo-encephalitis and is usually caused by type 2 (genital) herpes. In the encephalitis due to type 1 herpes simplex, the frontal and temporal lobes are primarily involved where there is a haemorrhagic necrosis. The CSF contains an increase in white cells and may be blood stained. CSF protein is raised but glucose is often normal. The EEG in this child shows characteristic features of herpes encephalitis, e.g. focal periodic slow waves over the frontal or temporal lobes. The CT scan may also show a focal abnormality. The diagnosis can only be confirmed by identifying the virus on brain biopsy. CSF titres which may take time to develop are not helpful.

Vidarabine, a nucleoside active against DNA viruses, has been shown to reduce the immediate mortality in herpes encephalitis, although the incidence of severe residual neurological defects was high. For treatment to be effective it must be given before permanent damage has occurred, and therefore started as early as possible. Acyclovir is an acyclic analogue of guanosine and only activated in infected cells. Its use in herpes encephalitis has recently been proven to be effective, and it is now the treatment of choice.

Further reading

MARSHALL, W. C. (1983) Infections of the nervous system. In *Paediatric Neurology*, edited by E. M. Brett, pp. 508–567. Edinburgh: Churchill Livingstone

WOOD, J. W. (1984) Antiviral chemotherapy. *Medicine International*, **2**, 102–104

Answer 86

Infant of diabetic mother.
Nesidioblastosis.
Islet cell adenoma.
Birth asphyxia.
Weidemann–Beckwith syndrome.
Leprechaunism (Donohue syndrome).
Hyperinsulinism in association with panhypopituitarism.
Severe rhesus incompatibility.

Discussion

Although the measurement of plasma insulin is not usually required in neonates who are hypoglycaemic, it is an important investigation in those where it is persistent or where excessive amounts of exogenous glucose are required for correction. Levels exceeding 10 mU/l when the blood glucose is <2.5 mmol/l are diagnostic of hyperinsulinism. This occurs commonly in infants of diabetic mothers, and is likely to be the case in this neonate whose birth weight is well above the 90th centile for gestation. Islet cell tissue is increased up to four-fold, due primarily to β-cell hyperplasia. The blood sugar can fall precipitously after delivery. Hypoglycaemia may be well tolerated, but symptoms such as lethargy and jitteriness may develop. Frank convulsions are associated with permanent neurological damage in approximately 50% of cases, but lesser symptoms result in permanent sequelae in 25%.

Birth asphyxia is also a relatively common cause of hyperinsulinism. Less commonly it may be due to nesidioblastosis (resulting from abnormal differentiation of the pancreatic islet cell tissue), islet cell adenoma, and Weidemann–Beckwith syndrome, severe rhesus incompatibility, Donohue syndrome, and in association with panhypopituitarism in the neonatal period. Weidemann–Beckwith syndrome is characterized by visceromegaly, macroglossia, exomphalos and gigantism. Thirty per cent of infants with this syndrome develop symptomatic hypoglycaemia in the neonatal period. Allthough this may be prolonged and severe it is more commonly transient.

Immediate treatment for all causes of hypoglycaemia is to maintain the blood glucose in the normal range. Infants with hyperinsulinism will require dextrose infusions, and rates of up to 20 mg/kg per min may be necessary. Intravenous hydrocortisone (5 mg/kg stat. followed by 1 mg/kg 6 hourly) is also commonly recommended for resistant cases. Glucagon may also be used. Diazoxide (15 mg/kg per day) inhibits insulin secretion, but may cause fluid retention. A thiazide diuretic (hydrochlorothiazide 5 mg/kg per day) potentiates the action of diazoxide and also reduces the fluid retention. In the case of nesidioblastosis, subtotal pancreatectomy is necessary for those not responding to medical treatment. In infants of diabetic mothers the insulin levels gradually return to normal.

Further reading

LEONARD, J. V. (1984) Recurrent post-neonatal hypoglycaemia. In *Chemical Pathology in the Sick Child*, edited by B. E. Clayton and J. M. Round, pp. 79–81. Oxford: Blackwell Scientific Publications

ROBERTON, N. R. C. (1986) Disorders of glucose homeostasis. *A Manual of Neonatal Intensive Care*, pp. 197–205. London: Edward Arnold

Answer 87

(1) Autosomal recessive
(2) 1 in 210.
(3) 1 in 8.

Discussion

The most likely pattern of inheritance is autosomal recessive – and this would be the expected answer. Autosomal dominant with impaired penetrance is possible, e.g. if one parent were subclinically affected and the gene is more fully expressed in the daughter.

Where the carriage rate is 1 in 35, the chances of two unaffected people meeting would be 1 in 1225 ($1/35 \times 1/35$) and the risk to their children would be 1 in 4900 ($1/35 \times 1/35 \times 1/4$).

When one parent has a chance of being a carrier then this calculation must be biased by the degree of risk of that person. In this situation that risk is two-thirds as the person is clinically normal. The risk of children would be 1 in 210 ($2/3 \times 1/35 \times 1/4$).

The risk to child B is harder to estimate because one has to estimate the carriage risks to her parents who are first cousins. The mother is definitely affected and will always pass on the gene. The father has a 1 in 4 chance of being a carrier as his mother has a 1 in 2 chance of being a carrier (because x and y must be carriers); combining the figures, the risks are 1 in 8 ($1/2 \times 1/1 \times 1/4$).

Answer 88

(1) Hypsarrhythmia.
(2) Infantile spasms.
(3) Perinatal asphyxia.
   Family history.
   Pertussis immunization.
   Previous developmental milestones.
(4) Blood sugar.
   Urine amino acids.
   Ophthalmological examination.
   Ultraviolet light examination.
   Developmental assessment.
   CT scan.

Discussion

The EEG shows the classical findings of hypsarrhythmia, namely high sharp single or multiple spikes interspersed by high voltage slow waves.

The clinical picture associated with hypsarrhythmia is one of infantile spasms – infantile myclonic seizures.

The majority are of unknown aetiology, but it is important to exclude treatable causes or conditions that have genetic implications – particularly the aminoacidopathies.

Infantile spasms are best classified into three main areas – initial investigation is orientated to differentiate each subgroup.

(1) Congenital causes
   Aircardi syndrome
   cerebral agenesis
   holoprosencephaly
   porencephaly.
   Investigation – CT scan.
(2) Metabolic causes
   aminoacidurias
   ceroid lipofuscinosis
   hypoglycaemia
   pyridoxine dependency
   Tay–Sachs disease.
   Investigation – urine amino acids, blood sugar, ophthalmological examination etc.
(3) Degenerative causes
   familial progressive myoclonic epilepsy
   incontinenti pigmenti
   Alper's disease
   Ramsay Hunt syndrome
   Sturge–Weber syndrome
   sudanophilic leucodystrophy
   tuberose sclerosis.

In addition to these main groups there are also: traumatic causes – anoxia or subdurals; toxic causes, e.g. antihistamines; and infectious causes, e.g. encephalitis or post-immunization.

The idiopathic group is where none of the above are evident. This group carries the best prognosis especially if the child is not developmentally delayed. Early treatment with ACTH is thought to offer the best prognosis.

Further reading

FORFAR, p. 817
NELSON, p. 1536

Answer 89

(1) The uptake and excretion by the left kidney appears normal. On the right there is poor function with a rising curve and persistence of activity at one hour.
(2) Severe right hydronephrosis.

Discussion

The normal renogram is divided into three phases:

(1) The vascular spike at about half a minute.
(2) Peak counts occur at about three and a half minutes, after which
(3) there is a gradual decline as isotope is cleared by the kidneys.

The curves from each kidney should be roughly symmetrical and of equal height. In this renogram the right side is obviously abnormal and excretion is delayed, suggesting an obstruction to urine output.

Further reading

BLAUFOX, D. M. and FREEMAN, L. M. (1973) Radionucleotide techniques for the evaluation of the urinary tract in children. *Seminars in Nuclear Medicine,* **3**, 27
GORDON, I. (1985) Imaging children with urinary tract infection. *Hospital Update,* **11**, 773

Answer 90

Atrial fibrillation.

Discussion

Atrial fibrillation can be recognized by the presence of fibrillatory waves (rate 400–700/min), the absence of P waves and the total irregularity of the ventricular response. In atrial flutter, by comparison, the atrial rate is 200–400/min and the ventricular rate usually regular.

Atrial fibrillation is rare in childhood, but can occur with a variety of structual heart defects, following cardiac surgery involving the atria, with severe mitral valve disease, or with myocardial disease. It may also be a complication of Wolff–Parkinson–White (WPW) syndrome, but in such a case it produces an irregular broad QRS tachycardia (looking like ventricular tachycardia).

Treatment for acute atrial fibrillation consists of DC external cardioversion or rapid digitalization. Digoxin is also the drug of choice in more chronic forms. DC cardioversion may be necessary, in which case digoxin should be discontinued for 24 hours beforehand. Disopyramide or amiodarone may help to maintain sinus rhythm. Anticoagulation is indicated in chronic atrial fibrillation prior to conversion to sinus rhythm, as left atrial thrombi can form. Chronic atrial fibrillation with underlying heart disease carries a poor prognosis.

Digoxin should be avoided in Wolf–Parkinson–White syndrome where it may facilitate conduction via the accessory pathway. Drugs that may be used for the Wolff–Parkinson–White syndrome with atrial fibrillation include flecainide, amiodarone or disopyramide.

Further reading

PARK, M. K. and GUNTHEROTH, W. G. (1981) *How to Read Pediatric ECGs.* Chicago: Year Book Medical Publishers Inc.

Answer 91

(1) Urinanalysis.
    Dextrostix or BM stix.
    Blood sugar.
(2) Diabetic ketoacidosis.

Discussion

The history of abdominal pain with a raised urea and hyponatraemia with serum osmolality within the normal range suggests a diagnosis of diabetic ketoacidosis. Glucose is osmotically active and, in excess, produces an osmotic gradient which draws water from the cells and causes hyponatraemia. The serum osmolality remains normal. Serum osmolality can be estimated by $2 \times [Na^+ + K^+] + glucose + urea$; therefore, in this case plasma glucose would be approximately 21 mmol/l. Urinanalysis and blood glucose estimation will confirm the diagnosis.

Non-hypotonic hyponatraemia also occurs in the 'sick cell syndrome', where the cells are thought to produce insufficient non-diffusible intracellular anions to maintain intracellular osmolality and also leak these anions into the plasma. Water diffuses out of the cells to maintain normal serum osmolality and hyponatraemia follows. In this case the actual serum osmolality remains normal, although the estimated serum osmolality will be low; there will therefore be an 'osmolal gap' (measured

– estimated osmolality). The sick cell syndrome occurs in severe illnesses such as septicaemia and liver failure.

Renal disease, such as the nephrotic syndrome, can also present with abdominal pain and hyponatraemia, but in such a case one would expect to find oedema, heavy proteinuria, and hypoalbuminaemia. The serum osmolality would be low.

Further reading

JAMIESON, M. J. (1985) Hyponatraemia. Clinical algorithms. *British Medical Journal*, **290**, 1723–1728

Answer 92

(1) Distal renal tubular acidosis.
(2) pH >6.
(3) Oral bicarbonate, 1–3 mmol/kg per day.

Discussion

This girl has a low plasma bicarbonate, hyperchloraemia and a normal anion gap, a combination seen in renal tubular acidosis (RTA). Nephrocalcinosis is rarely found in proximal renal tubular acidosis but is commonly associated with distal renal tubular acidosis. The water deprivation test shows she has a renal concentrating defect; the urine osmolality is well below that expected after fluid deprivation (>800 mosmol/kg). In both hypothalamic and nephrogenic diabetes insipidus the urine osmolality rarely exceeds 150 mosmol/kg, and neither of these conditions is associated with nephrocalcinosis. In distal renal tubular acidosis there is an inability to maintain a normal hydrogen ion gradient across the collecting duct, and this prevents the normal regeneration of bicarbonate. The loss of this important buffer increases the load on the other homeostatic systems: there is an excessive excretion of sodium and potassium salts in the urine and an increased resorption of bone with liberation of calcium and phosphate ions. Secondary hyperaldosteronism compounds the potassium loss.

Nephrocalcinosis results from calcium deposition in the interstitial medulla, and further damage is caused by the hypokalaemia. The effect of this damage is to decrease the concentrating ability of the kidneys and polyuria follows. The urine pH remains above 6 even in the face of severe acidosis. Treatment consists of small amounts of sodium bicarbonate (1–3 mmol/kg per day), less than is needed in proximal renal tubular acidosis. Potassium supplementation may also be necessary.

Other causes of medullary nephrocarcinosis include primary hyperparathyroidism, sarcoidosis, milk–alkali syndrome, primary hyperoxaluria and idiopathic hypercalciuria. Primary hypoparathyroidism is excluded by the normal calcium level.

Further reading

MORRIS, R. C. and SEBASTIAN, A. (1983) Renal tubular acidosis and the Fanconi syndrome. In *The Metabolic Basis of Inherited Disease,* edited by J. B. Stanbury, J. B. Wyngaarden, D. S. Fredrickson, J. L. Goldstein and M. S. Brown, pp. 1803–1843. New York: McGraw-Hill Book Company
NELSON, pp. 1344–1347

Answer 93

(1) Minimum age two and a half.
(2) The child has a physical or neurological lesion affecting both legs.

Discussion

This question is taken almost directly from the Denver Developmental Screening Test (DDST). The first three pieces of information are taken from the hearing and speech section – the 25th centile for passing these items is two and three-quarter years. Taking two and a half years as a minimum age therefore seems reasonable.

Sitting unsupported and being unable to walk puts the child between 8 and 11 months for posture – there is no information regarding arm movements but one must presume the child has normal arms to allow support reactions while sitting.

There is a marked discrepancy between the locomotor abilities and higher functions in this child and the interpretation is that the child probably has a neurological lesion affecting the legs – this could be a spastic diplegia, spina bifida or similar lesion.

Answer 94

(1) Hyperoxia.
   Mixed metabolic/respiratory acidosis.
   Low white blood cell count.
   Low platelet count.
(2) Full infection screen.
(3) Decrease inspired oxygen concentration.
   Give fresh frozen plasma.
   Treat with antibiotics.

Discussion

This neonate has, apart from the platelet count, 'normal' coagulation indices for his degree of prematurity and birth weight (control values will be from adults or older children). Treatment is, however, required to prevent further bleeding either into the skin or internally. Vitamin K is unlikely to have any significant effect upon the immature liver; thawed fresh frozen plasma should be given intravenously.

Platelet numbers are not normally low in premature infants, although a count of $80 \times 10^9/l$ will not in itself cause bleeding. The WBC is also significantly reduced; this and thrombocytopenia both raise the possibility of infection, necessitating investigation and broad spectrum intravenous antibiotic therapy.

The arterial blood gas shows a slightly low bicarbonate, indicative of a mild metabolic acidosis, but with a raised CO_2. There is, therefore, a mixed metabolic/respiratory acidosis. Neither of these are unexpected for an infant of this gestation and are compatible with respiratory distress syndrome.

Treatment with sodium bicarbonate is only indicated for severe acidosis; in any event a respiratory acidosis with a raised CO_2 requires measures to improve gaseous exchange. Since the CO_2 is not very high, and, providing the infant is otherwise stable, no change in ventilation would be necessary; however, the arterial oxygen concentration is too high and the inspired oxygen needs to be decreased.

Further reading

FORFAR, pp. 191–194
KLAUS, M. H. and FANAROFF, A. A. (1979) *Care of the High Risk Neonate*. Philadelphia: W. B. Saunders
ROBERTON, N. R. C. (1986) *A Manual of Neonatal Intensive Care*. London: Edward Arnold

Answer 95

(1) X-linked agammaglobulinaemia.
(2) Reduction in placentally transmitted IgG.

Discussion

In this boy low levels of IgG, IgA and IgM are accompanied by abnormalities in B-cell function and number. Neutrophil and total lymphocyte counts are normal. Defective B-cell function is evident by the absence of isohaemagglutinins (IgM antibodies found in >90% of children by 1 year who are not blood group AB) and of surface membrane immunoglobulins.

T-cell lymphocytes are identified by their ability to form rosettes with sheep red blood cells, and the result is expressed as a percentage of total lymphocyte numbers. In the absence of B cells this percentage will be increased. Monoclonal antibodies are also used for identifying and characterizing T lymphocytes. Those directed against the T_3 receptor give a measure of total T-cell numbers, those against the T_4 receptor, helper–inducer cell numbers and those against the T_8 receptor, suppressor/cytotoxic cell numbers.

The response to the mitogen phytohaemagglutinin (PHA) is a measure of T-cell proliferation. The nitroblue tetrazolium (NBT) dye reduction test is an *in vitro* measure of granulocyte function; in all individuals apart from those who have chronic granulomatous disease, or those who are carriers for this disorder, over 98% of granulocytes take up NBT and reduce it from yellow to blue.

Thus the data given here indicate an isolated B-cell deficiency. The age of onset in this boy and the family history strongly suggest a diagnosis of X-linked agammaglobulinaemia (Bruton's disease.) Children with this disorder are protected in the first months of life by maternal IgG transmitted across the placenta, but as levels fall they become susceptible to pyogenic infections. Treatment consists of repeated immunoglobulin injections. Other causes of hypogammaglobulinaemia include common variable hypogammaglobulinaemia of childhood, hypogammaglobulinaemia with raised IgM levels (usually X-linked) and transient deficiency of infancy.

Further reading

FORFAR, pp. 1340–1341
HAYWARD, A. R. (1983) Specific immunodeficiency. In *Paediatric Immunology*, edited by J. F. Soothill, A. R. Hayward and C. B. S. Wood, pp. 156–211. Oxford: Blackwell Scientific Publications
NELSON, pp. 1340–1341

Answer 96

(1) Peak expiratory flow rate; vital capacity measurement; lumbar puncture; nerve conduction studies.
(2) Guillain–Barré syndrome.
(3) Generally good.

Discussion

Vital capacity and peak expiratory flow rate (PEFR) are the most important investigations from a practical point of view – respiratory failure is the cause of death in this condition.

Lumbar puncture is useful after the first week of symptoms; it characteristically shows a raised protein and a minor lymphocytosis, but this may not be present in the first week.

Both motor and sensory nerve conduction studies are slow.

The pointers toward the diagnosis of Guillain–Barré syndrome are:

(1) The symmetrical loss including proximal and distal muscle groups.
(2) Sensory involvement – distal limb and autonomic.
(3) Cranial nerve involvement (VII is the commonest).
(4) Loss of joint sensation leading to apparent ataxia.

No preceding viral infection is seen in 25%.
Differential diagnosis should include:

(1) Poliomyelitis (CSF cells increased, no sensory involvement, often unilateral).
(2) Spinal cord tumour (no signs above the lesion, progressive upper motor neurone signs) – sphincters often involved.
(3) Polymyositis (no sensory changes and creatine phosphokinase elevated).
(4) Cerebellar disorder – weakness, hypotonia and incoordination.

Outcome is generally good with ventilatory support and physiotherapy. However, some go on to a relapsing course and a few chronically progress. Having progressed to a maximum of weakness, symptoms remain static for a period of time before improvement begins. The longer the static period, especially after 16 days, the more likely is incomplete recovery.

Further reading

BRETT E. M. (Ed.) (1983) *Paediatric Neurology*. Edinburgh: Churchill Livingstone
FORFAR, pp. 799, 847
NELSON, p. 1603

Answer 97

(1) Phenobarbitone/phenytoin overdose.
(2) History, and anticonvulsant levels.

Discussion

Cerebellar ataxia is rare in children.

Drug overdose must be high on the list of differential diagnoses for acute cerebellar ataxia and, therefore, a careful history orientated toward all the medicines/illnesses in the family should be taken. Other agents causing ataxia include alcohol, minor tranquillizers, bromides, 5-fluorouracil and DDT.

Where there are signs of systemic upset an encephalitis primarily affecting the cerebellum should be considered, i.e. acute cerebritis – usually there is a raised CSF white cell count, normal glucose and late rise in CSF protein.

Prolonged hyperthermia associated with other systemic illnesses can produce a self-limiting cerebellar ataxia.

Cerebellar concussion following trauma also needs to be considered.

Post-infectious cerebellar ataxias do occur (similar to Guillain–Barré syndrome but affecting the cerebellum), but usually there is an element of weakness. Chickenpox is the commonest cause. A specific syndrome has been recognized consisting of ataxia, areflexia and ophthalmoplegia (Fisher's syndrome) which appears to be a separate entity from Guillain–Barré syndrome.

Chronic ataxias in childhood are too numerous to mention but their main groupings are metabolic, toxic, congenital, endocrine, neoplastic, vascular and degenerative.

Further reading

FORFAR, pp. 719, 724
SWANMAN, K. F. and WRIGHT, F. S. (1982) *The Practice of Pediatric Neurology*, 2nd edn. New York: C. V. Mosby

Answer 98

(1) Infectious mononucleosis.
(2) Paul–Bunnell test.
(3) Platelet count.
(4) Ask about contact with ampicillin.

Discussion

Infectious mononucleosis generally presents with lymphadenopathy, often with an exudative tonsillitis (30%), splenomegaly (50%) and hepatomegaly (30%).

A rash may be seen in 10% but the 'ampicillin rash' is almost diagnostic (it also occurs with cytomegalovirus).

Rarer presentations include hepatitis, thrombocytopenia, haemolytic anaemia, encephalitis and Guillain–Barré syndrome.

This child has a mild haemolytic anaemia (low haemoglobin, raised reticulocyte count – presuming no recent blood loss), a sore throat, a rash and a typical white blood cell count. Most patients have 25% atypical mononuclear cells by the second and third week of their illness.

The Paul–Bunnell test relies on the presence of a heterophile antibody to sheep red cells that is absorbed by beef red cells but not guinea-pig kidney cells. Titres of 1/52 and greater are significant. It is less likely to be positive in the young child.

Other causes of a monocytosis include:

(1) Chronic bacterial infections, e.g. tuberculosis, brucellosis, endocarditis, typhoid.
(2) Protozoan diseases.
(3) Chronic neutropenia.
(4) Hodgkin's disease.
(5) Myelocytic and monocytic leukaemia.

Further reading

HOFFBRAND, A. V. and PETTIT, J. E. (1984) *Essential Haematology,* p. 99. Oxford: Blackwell Scientific
WILLOUGHBY, M. L. N. (1977) *Paediatric Haematology,* p. 244. Edinburgh: Churchill

Answer 99

(1) Ornithine carbamoyl transferase deficiency (OCTD).
(2) Yes: X-linked inheritance but females can be affected.

Discussion

A serum ammonia of 200 µmol/l is well above the normal range (<40 µmol/l). Acute encephalopathy with hyperammonaemia suggests a diagnosis of Reye's syndrome, but previous illnesses associated with drowsiness and the death of a male sibling make a diagnosis of ornithine carbamoyl transferase deficiency more likely. This is the most common of the urea cycle disorders and has an X-linked inheritance. Affected males usually develop a severe encephalopathy and die in the neonatal period. Female heterozygotes may be completely asymptomatic or may have a characteristic episodic or fluctuating illness often associated with viral infections. A urea cycle disorder should always be considered in those children who have had recurrent encephalopathic illnesses or a second attack of a Reye's-like illness.

Orotic acid excretion is increased in the urine and this can be used to identify asymptomatic carriers following a standard protein load.

The diagnosis of ornithine carbamoyl transferase deficiency can be confirmed by enzyme assay in liver tissue.

Other rare urea cycle disorders include carbamoyl phosphate synthetase deficiency, arginosuccinate synthetase deficiency, arginosuccinate lyase deficiency, arginase deficiency and *N*-acetyl glutamate synthetase deficiency.

Serum ammonia is not always easily measured in many hospitals. The level is falsely raised if the sample is allowed to haemolyse or clot and the analysis must be completed shortly after collection.

It should be remembered that convulsions in children are common and only rarely due to inherited metabolic disorder.

Further reading

LEONARD, J. V. (1984) Hyperammonaemia in childhood. In *Chemical Pathology in the Sick Child,* edited by B. E. Clayton and J. M. Round, pp. 96–119. Oxford: Blackwell Scientific Publications
WALSER, M. (1983) Urea cycle disorders and other hereditary hyperammonemic syndromes. In *The Metabolic Basis of Inherited Diseases,* edited by J. B. Stanbury, J. B. Wyngaarden, D. S. Fredrickson, J. L. Goldstein and M. S. Brown, pp. 402–437. New York: McGraw-Hill Book Company

Answer 100

Supraventricular tachycardia.

Discussion

Paroxysmal supraventricular tachycardia (SVT) is the commonest tachyarrhythmia in childhood. In over 70% of cases the heart is normal, the remaining 30% usually being associated with diseases of the myocardium, atrial septal defect or Ebstein's anomaly. Supraventricular tachycardia arises from either increased automaticity of cells within the atria, AV junction or His–Purkinje system, or, as in the majority of cases, from re-entry.

Supraventricular tachycardia can usually be identified on the ECG by finding a regular ventricular rate, above 180 beats/min, with a normal QRS complex. In some cases, however, one of the bundle-branches is refractory when the impulse reaches the AV node and a QRS pattern resembling bundle-branch block occurs. This can sometimes make it difficult to differentiate supraventricular tachycardia from a ventricular arrhythmia. If P waves are seen they are regular, with a rate of 200–400/min.

ST depression is often associated with paroxysmal supraventricular tachycardia and may remain present for up to 24 hours following attacks.

In this ECG the ventricular rate is approximately 210 beats/min and regular. The QRS complex is not prolonged although there is a degree of terminal slurring in AVR, V1, V2 and V4R. There is ST depression in V2, V4 and V6. P waves are not seen.

Brief, infrequent, asymptomatic attacks of paroxysmal supraventricular tachycardia do not usually require treatment, but prolonged episodes may lead to heart failure, especially in infants. Underlying causes, such as hypoxia, electrolyte disturbances, digoxin toxicity etc. should be identified and corrected if possible. Vagal stimulation may abort some attacks. Drugs used to induce sinus rhythm include digoxin, propranolol, verapamil and disopyramide (verapamil should never be used in combination with a β-blocker). Synchronized cardioversion is frequently successful, but must be performed under sedation or general anaesthesia. Digoxin ± β-blockers are useful for reducing the frequency of attacks.

Further reading

FORFAR, pp. 658–661
JORDON, S. C. and SCOTT, O. (1981) *Heart Disease in Paediatrics*, 2nd edn, pp. 298–303. London: Butterworths

Answer 101

(1) Turner's syndrome.
(2) Chromosome analysis.

Discussion

In this girl basal LH and FSH levels are very high, whereas the plasma oestradiol level is low. These findings are diagnostic of gonadal dysgenesis. Her height is below the third centile for age. This combination of short stature, gonadal dysgenesis and coarctation suggests the diagnosis of Turner's syndrome. Coarctation of the aorta is the commonest cardiac lesion in this condition and osteoporosis is characteristic of patients who are not diagnosed until their teens.

Although Turner's syndrome can usually be diagnosed clinically, this is not always the case, particularly when there is only a partial absence of a sex chromosome. In the majority of cases of Turner's syndrome, chromosomal analysis shows a karyotype of 45XO, but in the remainder there is mosaicism, partial deletion or an isochromosome or ring chromosome present and the clinical picture may be modified. In Noonan's syndrome no chromosomal abnormality can be detected, but cardiac lesions usually involve the pulmonary artery or valve.

Further reading

BROOK, C. G. D. (1986) Turner syndrome. *Archives of Disease in Childhood*, **61**, 305–309
CHAUSSAIN, J. L. (1981) Late puberty. In *Clinical Paediatric Endocrinology*, edited by C. G. D. Brook, pp. 240–247. Oxford: Blackwell Scientific Publications
VISSER, H. K. A. (1984) Precocious and delayed puberty. In *Chemical Pathology in the Sick Child*, edited by B. E. Clayton and J. M. Round, pp. 343–364. Oxford: Blackwell Scientific Publications

Answer 102

(1) Haemolytic uraemic syndrome.
(2) Blood pressure.
    Urine output.

Discussion

Haemolytic anaemia with fragmented red cells, thrombocytopenia and renal failure fulfils the diagnostic criteria for haemolytic uraemic syndrome. The prodromal illnesses of diarrhoea and vomiting are classically seen in the epidemic form of this disease. This boy has neurological involvement, most likely due to hypertensive encephalopathy although it could also be secondary to electrolyte disturbance or caused by microthrombi. It is, therefore, important to know the blood pressure and treat as appropriate, remembering that cerebral perfusion pressure is a function of systemic blood pressure and intercranial pressure: lowering the blood pressure to normal levels without adequately treating coexisting raised intercranial pressure may be disastrous.

Haemolytic uraemic syndrome can be divided into two distinct groups. The first, an epidemic form, occurs primarily in infants in the summer and is associated with a good prognosis with supportive treatment alone. The second, a sporadic form, is not associated with a prodromal illness and affects older children. The predisposition to the disease in this group appears to be inherited as an autosomal recessive trait. The prognosis is much poorer with irreversible renal failure a common outcome. Renal damage in the epidemic group is primarily glomerular with a thrombotic microangiopathy, but in the sporadic group is arteriolar with intimal and subintimal oedema, necrosis and proliferation.

The cause of this heterogenous disorder is not known, but a variety of bacteria and viruses have been implicated at various times. Clotting studies are usually normal or near normal and the hypothesis that haemolytic uraemic syndrome is associated with an abnormal activation of the clotting system has not been confirmed. The prostaglandin PGI_2, produced by the endothelial cells, is known to be important in preventing thrombosis. Abnormalities of PGI_2 metabolism appear to be associated at least with the sporadic group. These include inhibition of PGI_2 synthesis, increased degradation of PGI_2, and deficiency of a plasma factor necessary for PGI_2 production. The presence of platelet aggregating factors has also been found in some patients in this group. The majority of these patients have required plasmaphoresis to induce remission. Endothelial toxins may be the cause of the epidemic form in which abnormalities of PGI_2 are not characteristic.

Further reading

FONG, S. C., DE-CHADAREVIAN, J. and KAPLAN, B. S. (1982) Haemolytic-uraemic syndrome: current concepts and management. *Paediatric Clinics of North America*, **29**, 835–836

LEVIN, M. and BARRATT, T. M. (1984) Haemolytic uraemic syndrome. *Archives of Disease in Childhood*, **59**, 397–400

Answer 103

(1) Metabolic acidosis with partial respiratory compensation.
(2) Blood pressure.
(3) Sepsis – group B streptococcal disease.
(4) Congenital heart disease.
    Inborn errors of metabolism.

Discussion

With this degree of metabolic acidosis, cardiac output starts to be compromised; blood pressure is often overlooked in neonatal examination – it is particularly relevant in this situation.

The group B streptococcus is very sensitive to penicillin and, unless this diagnosis is considered early, the condition may be rapidly fatal.

Structural congenital heart disease leading to low cardiac output leads to poor tissue perfusion and resulting metabolic acidosis.

Inborn errors of metabolism are considered, particularly if the acidosis is resistant to therapy or recurs after the reintroduction of feeds.

Further reading

FORFAR, pp. 136, 143

Answer 104

(1) Toxocara infection.
(2) Serology for *Toxocara* or toxocara skin test.
(3) Advice on hygiene and deworming of pets.

Discussion

The clinical description is classical – *Toxocara* is the only helminth affecting the eyes in temperate climates; he has had recurrent bouts of bronchitis and even his enuresis might be due to encystment in the bladder. He is a little underweight and slightly anaemic.

Investigation reveals eosinophilia and examination an enlarged liver.

The serological test used is either indirect fluorescent antibody or an ELISA assay.

Both the serology and the skin test may be negative where there is a limited infection and so liver biopsy would provide the definitive diagnosis.

His parents need information about transmission and advice on general hygiene. The children should avoid play areas where dogs defaecate and their own dogs should be dewormed regularly.

Further reading

FORFAR, pp. 1501, 1507
NELSON, p. 859

Answer 105

(1) He has a haemolytic anaemia – due to vitamin E deficiency.
(2) Cystic fibrosis.
(3) Sweat test.

Discussion

The pointers toward the diagnosis are an infant who is feeding well, but not gaining weight, though not all infants with cystic fibrosis do feed well. Investigations suggest malabsorption (hypoalbuminaemia) and the chest X-ray shows two areas of consolidation.

The haemolytic anaemia, suggested by the reticulocyte count and raised bilirubin, is rare but well recognized in cystic fibrosis.

Causes of a false positive sweat test include:

Adrenal insufficiency
Flucloxacillin therapy
Ectodermal dysplasia
Nephrogenic diabetes insipidus
Fucosidosis
Mucopolysaccharidoses
Hypothyroidism
Glucose-6-phosphatase deficiency
Glycogen storage disease (type I)
Salt loading during the neonatal period.

Further reading

FORFAR, p. 511
NELSON, p. 1086

Answer 106

Glycogen storage disease.

Discussion

Hypoglycaemia and hyperlipidaemia occur in both type I and type III glycogen storage disease, but very high cholesterol levels are usually only found in type I glycogen storage disease (normal range: serum triglyceride, 0.35–1.0 mmol/l, serum cholesterol, 3.0–5.5 mmol/l).

Type Ia glycogen storage disease (von Gierke's disease) is due to deficiency of glucose-6-phosphatase. Children may present in the neonatal period with acidosis and hypoglycaemia, or later in early infancy with hepatomegaly and failure to thrive. Although hypoglycaemic convulsions are not uncommon, the low blood glucose is well tolerated with ketones used as an alternative fuel. Hyperuricaemia and bleeding also occur. Mental development is normal. There is little or no rise in blood glucose with subcutaneous glucagon or adrenaline, nor any increase following intravenous fructose or galactose, both of which may produce acidosis. The diagnosis is confirmed by assay of glucose-6-phosphatase in the liver.

In type Ib (pseudo type I) there is normal *in-vitro* activity of glucose-6-phosphatase, but a defect in its microsomal transport. Clinically, both types Ia and Ib present in the same manner but, in the latter, there is also an abnormality in both neutrophil function and numbers. Infection in these children is a major problem, adversely affecting their prognosis.

In type III glycogen storage disease there is deficiency of amylo-1,6-glucosidase, the enzyme responsible for degradation of glycogen at its branch points. This disease is clinically similar to type I glycogen storage disease but less severe. Subcutaneous or intravenous glucagon causes a rise in blood glucose after a meal but not during fasting. Galactose can be converted normally to glucose.

Further reading

FORFAR, pp. 1251–1257
HOWELL, R. R. and WILLIAMS, J. C. (1983) The glycogen storage diseases. In *The Metabolic Basis of Inherited Diseases*, edited by J. B. Stanbury, J. B. Wyngaarden, D. S. Fredrickson, J. L. Goldstein and M. S. Brown, pp. 141–166. New York: McGraw-Hill Book Company
NELSON, pp. 455–466

Answer 107

(1) No peak in middle ear compliance.
(2) Perforation.
    Completely fluid-filled middle ear.
(3) External auditory canal volume.

Discussion

This illustrates how tympanograms should not be read in isolation from other data. Two very dissimilar conditions give identical traces.

With perforation there is no build-up of pressure in the external auditory canal because there is a free connection with the atmosphere (via the perforation and the eustachian tube).

There is no change in mobility of the tympanic membrane because fluid in the middle ear is non-compressible and, therefore, the mobility of the drum remains the same despite pressure changes. The result is a horizontal line.

The external auditory canal volume would be normal in the latter condition of fluid-filled middle ear but infinite in the former condition of perforation (i.e. unrecordable).

Answer 108

(1) Protein losing enteropathy.
(2) Chromium-labelled albumin studies.

Discussion

Hypoalbuminaemia, not accounted for by proteinuria, with a history of diarrhoea suggests the diagnosis.
  Protein losing enteropathy may be secondary to:

(1) Defective lymphatic drainage of the gut, e.g. intestinal lymphangiectasia, thoracic duct obstruction or even cardiac failure.
(2) Inflammatory bowel conditions – Crohn's disease or ulcerative colitis, tuberculosis.
(3) Unknown mechanisms – coeliac disease, cystic fibrosis, food allergy – which disrupt the balance of turnover in the gut (15% of albumin and globulin turnover is accounted for in the gut).

^{51}Cr-labelled albumin techniques demonstrate increased gut losses.
  Lymphocyte count may be reduced in states due to lymphatic obstruction. Additional investigation of the gastrointestinal tract including intestinal biopsy will be indicated to elucidate the underlying cause of the protein loss.

Further reading

ANDERSON, C. M. and BURKE, V. (1975) *Paediatric Gastroenterology*, p. 273. Oxford: Blackwell Scientific
FORFAR, pp. 462, 1231
NELSON, p. 511

Answer 109

(1) Ventilation–perfusion mismatch.
(2) Post-traumatic pulmonary arteriovenous fistula.
(3) Radioisotope perfusion scan.

Discussion

The lung function tests are normal yet at rest he is hypoxic – resulting in secondary polycythaemia. Presuming no structural heart disease, then a pulmonary arteriovenous fistula must have developed.

Answer 110

(1) Decreased right and left heart saturations.
    Increased right and left ventricular end-diastolic pressures.
    Increased pulmonary artery pressure.
    Increased V-wave pressure.
(2) Congestive heart failure.

Discussion

In this boy, decreased right heart oxygen saturations are indicative of reduced cardiac output, decreased saturations from the pulmonary artery to the aorta suggest pulmonary oedema and increased end-diastolic pressures and moderately raised pulmonary artery pressure confirm the presence of biventricular failure. The increased V-wave pressure is a consequence of mitral regurgitation associated with left ventricular dilatation.

Children with cardiomyopathies are rarely catheterized as the diagnosis can be made on echo alone.

The cause of congestive cardiomyopathy in childhood is usually unknown. In some cases it is familial and in others there may be a history of viral infection.

The onset is often insidious and the disease progressive, with a poor prognosis, although occasionally some children make a full recovery. Death may be caused by intractable heart failure, or arrhythmias. Intracardiac thrombosis may cause systemic emboli.

Treatment with digoxin and diuretics is indicated for cardiac failure. Prednisolone has been used in progressive cases although it has not been shown to be effective.

Further reading

JORDON, S. C. and SCOTT, O. (1981) *Heart Disease in Paediatrics*, 2nd edn, pp. 321–338. London: Butterworths
NELSON, pp. 1186–1189
ROSSI, E. (1983) Cardiomyopathy in infancy. *Modern Problems in Paediatrics*, **22**, 15–25

Answer 111

(1) Pineal tumour.
(2) Skull X-ray.
    CT scan.

Discussion

Midbrain compression by a tumour in the pineal area causes loss of conjugate eye movements and pupillary dilatation with reduction in the light reflex (a combination known as Parinaud's syndrome). For pineal tumours 10–15% are associated with precocious puberty in males.

In this child the bone age is significantly advanced, testicular volume is 18 ml (prepubertal level <4 ml) and the LHRH stimulation test shows a high basal LH level and pubertal FSH response. Skull X-rays often show pineal calcification and this, in children, is very suggestive of a tumour.

Pinealomas are rare under the age of 12 years but are more common in males (M:F, 9:1). Other tumours in this region include teratomas, hamartomas and astrocytomas. The treatment of choice is partial surgical removal followed by irradiation. Total surgical removal is technically difficult and associated with a high mortality. A shunt procedure for hydrocephalus followed by radiotherapy may be needed. The long-term outlook is poor.

Further reading

BRETT, E. M. (ed.) (1983) Intracranial and spinal cord lesions. In *Paediatric Neurology*, pp. 430–461. Edinburgh: Churchill Livingstone

GIRARD, J. (1983) Intracranial space-occupying lesions. In *Clinical Paediatric Endocrinology*, edited by C. G. D. Brook, pp. 275–284 Oxford: Blackwell Scientific Publications

Answer 112

(1) Type II respiratory failure.
(2) Hypoventilation.
(3) Mechanical ventilation.

Discussion

Type I respiratory failure, when hypoxaemia (Po_2 <10 kPa) is found in combination with a low Pco_2, can occur, for example, with pulmonary oedema, asthma, pneumonia and pulmonary embolism. Hyperventilation is caused by stimulation of pulmonary afferents and this leads to a fall in the Pco_2. Type II respiratory failure is seen with disorders that result in hypoventilation. In this case there is hypoxaemia and hypercapnia (Pco_2 >6 kPa). Hypoventilation may be caused by an abnormality in ventilatory control with depression of the respiratory centre (e.g. due to head injury, drugs etc.), or by diseases limiting thoracic movement (e.g. kyphoscoliosis), respiratory muscle disease, or neural or neuromuscular disease. It may also occur in severe asthma or pneumonia, in respiratory obstruction, pneumothorax and pleurisy.

Respiratory failure from paralysis of the intercostal muscles is the most serious complication of post-infectious polyneuritis (Guillain–Barré syndrome). Frequent assessment of respiratory function is necessary in this disease and assisted ventilation started before respiratory failure becomes advanced. Over 90% of children eventually recover but ventilation may be necessary for several weeks or even months.

This girl has type II respiratory failure and is acidotic. She therefore requires assisted ventilation urgently.

Further reading

BRETT, E. M. (Ed.) (1983) *Paediatric Neurology*, pp. 118–122. Edinburgh: Churchill Livingstone
FLENLEY, C. F. (1982) Respiratory function tests. *Medicine International*, **1**, 937

Answer 113

(1) Iron deficiency anaemia.
(2) Serum ferritin or serum iron and total iron binding capacity.
Haemoglobin electrophoresis.

Discussion

The differentiation of iron deficiency and β-thalassaemia trait is often difficult using red cell indices only; indeed because iron deficiency is so common the two conditions may well coexist.

The following formula may be helpful:

$$DF = MCV - RBC - (5 \times Hb) - 3.4$$

If the DF (discriminant function) is positive then iron deficiency is present, when negative β-thalassaemia trait is present. The formula is not valid in haemodilute states, e.g. post-haemorrhage or pregnancy.

This child has a positive value and it is inferred that he or she is iron deficient – the correct course of action would be to prescribe a course of iron therapy and then review the indices. It is possible that recalculation of the discriminant function would now have a negative value indicating β-thalassaemia, i.e. the iron deficiency was having the greater effect and, now corrected, the β-thalassaemia trait is evident.

The majority of children with β-thalassaemia trait have raised HbA_2 levels (3.4–7.0%), a small number show high HbF levels but haemoglobin electrophoresis will identify both groups.

If thalassaemia trait is diagnosed it is important to provide accurate genetic advice – which will require testing of parents and other siblings.

Further reading

ADDY, D. P. (1986) Happiness is: Iron. *British Medical Journal*, **292**, 969
ENGLAND, J. M. and FRASER, P. M. (1973) Differentiation of iron deficiency from thalassaemia trait by routine blood count. *Lancet*, **i**, 449
NELSON, p. 1227

Answer 114

(1) Ataxia telangiectasia.
(2) Telangiectasia of the bulbar conjuctivae.
(3) Serum α-fetoprotein.
    CT brain scan.
    Chest tomograms.
    Radiation sensitivity of cultured leucocytes and fibroblasts.

Discussion

The combination of ataxia, very low IgA, low or absent IgE and recurrent infections is seen in ataxia telangiectasia, a neurodermatosis inherited as an autosomal recessive character. Children with this condition tend to be late in walking, and hyptonic. Ataxia develops slowly until there is frank choreoathetosis, defects in conjugate eye movements and severe dysarthria.

Telangiectasia of the bulbar conjunctivae is usually evident by 5 years of age. This spreads to the nasolabial folds, the ears, and along the flexor creases of the elbows and knees. Deterioration is usually gradual; most children are wheelchair bound by their early teens with death from respiratory infection and malnutrition following within a few years.

Immunological defects consist of low or absent IgA and IgE and hypoplasia of the thymus with abnormal cellular immunity. Delayed hypersensitivity reactions, as demonstrated by intradermal injection of candida antigens, are reduced or absent. Recurrent chest, ear and sinus infections may occur, although the susceptibility to these is variable. There is also an increased incidence of malignancy, particularly medulloblastomas and lymphomas.

Serum levels of α-fetoprotein are raised. Other investigations that might also be helpful include tomograms of the chest (small thymic shadow) and a CT brain scan (small cerebellum). Cultured leucocytes and fibroblasts may show characteristically abnormal radiation sensitivity.

The differential diagnosis is from other forms of ataxia, particularly the ataxic form of cerebral palsy which can be very similar before the development of telangiectasia in ataxia telangiectasia. Freidreich's ataxia is usually of later onset. Telangiectasia is also seen in the Sturge–Weber syndrome.

Further reading

CAVANAGH, N. (1979) *A Scheme of Paediatric Neurological Investigation.* Geigy Pharmaceuticals

HAYWARD, A. R. (1983) Specific immunodeficiency. In *Paediatric Immunology*, edited by J. F. Soothill, A. R. Hayward and C. B. S. Wood, pp. 156–211. Oxford: Blackwell Scientific Publications

Answer 115

(1) Partially treated bacterial meningitis.
(2) CSF cultures.
    Blood cultures.
    Counter-immunoelectrophoresis.
    Viral cultures.
    Ziehl–Nielsen stain.

Discussion

A low CSF glucose with raised protein is evidence of CSF infection. In viral meningitis CSF glucose is generally normal, although this is not always true, particularly in mumps meningitis. Tuberculous meningitis could be consistent with these results but the short history and initial response to antibiotics is against this diagnosis. Organisms are often not seen in partially treated meningitis and there may be a mixed polymorph lymphocytic or monocytic response. Fragmented cells may also be present.

Counter-immunoelectrophoresis (CIE) is a rapid method of detecting bacterial antigens in either urine or CSF. False negative results do occur and it should not be relied upon to exclude bacterial infection. Blood and/or CSF may be sterile with prior antibiotic administration although, as in this boy, deterioration is more likely to be associated with positive cultures.

Further reading

MARSHALL, W. C. (1983) Infections of the nervous system. In *Paediatric Neurology*, edited by E. M. Brett, pp. 508–567. Edinburgh: Churchill Livingstone

Answer 116

(1) Pulmonary hypertension.
    Right heart failure (cor pulmonale).
(2) Oxygen.

Discussion

The blood gases show a reduced pH and arterial Po_2 without a rise in Pco_2.

The ECG is reported as showing peaked P waves in leads II, III and aVF and changes of RVH in the chest leads. The P wave changes are indicative of chronically increased central venous pressure and right atrial hypertrophy.

Chronic hypoxia leads to increasing pulmonary arterial muscle tone. Usually this would shunt blood to areas of lung better aerated but, where lung function is poor throughout, the result is pulmonary hypertension, leading in turn to right heart failure.

Untreated secondary infection could also lead to deterioration in symptoms and these blood gas changes.

Initially the changes of pulmonary artery tone are reversible with oxygen. Attention should also be paid to appropriate antibiotic therapy given intravenously and to the frequency and technique of chest physiotherapy.

Answer 117

(1) ABO incompatibility.
    Rhesus incompatibility (anti-E).
    Other less common blood group incompatibilities (e.g. Kell).
(2) Yes.
(3) Serial bilirubin estimation.
    Haemoglobin.
    Reticulocyte count.
    Phototherapy or exchange transfusion if required.
    Observe for late anaemia.

Discussion

The homozygous combination CDe/CDe occurs in approximately 16% of the Caucasian population; the genotype of the infant is not given so it would be possible to inherit a rhesus gene from the father.

There is more chance of 'small' genotype incompatibility producing a clinical problem when the mother and infant are not ABO incompatible – the fetal cells have a greater chance of survival and can therefore induce antibody production.

Most minor blood group incompatibilities are not serious – however, this cannot be predicted and therefore all jaundiced infants require serial bilirubin estimations until the individual trend is established. Where considerable haemolysis has occurred *in utero* the haemoglobin will be low and the reticulocyte count raised.

Answer 118

(1) Generalized spikes and waves at a frequency of nearly 3 Hz (cycles per second).
(2) 'Absences' – typical of petit mal – the child momentarily loses consciousness but not posture.
(3) Overbreathing or rapid blinking. (In the laboratory flashing lights may be used.)

Answer 119

(1) Hypoglycaemic convulsion.
(2) 'Septic screen'.
    Urine reducing substances.
(3) Intravenous 10% dextrose.
    Antibiotics.

Discussion

Apnoeic episodes may be the presenting feature of many pathologies in the newborn period. The data presented show hypoglycaemia. A generalized convulsion in the neonate may not have a clonic component, merely the tonic, or apnoeic, part.

Having established hypoglycaemia as the likely cause of the apnoea, investigation is directed at explaining the hypoglycaemia.

Infection is the most likely explanation in an otherwise full-grown term delivery. A full infection screen must therefore be performed.

The minimum infection screen should include blood cultures, CSF examination, urine culture and chest X-ray.

Galactosaemia is rare (1:50 000) but should be considered because, if left untreated, it leads to mental retardation.

Further reading

FORFAR, pp. 231, 1188
NELSON, pp. 447, 964

Answer 120

(1) Left and right atrial hypertrophy.
    Marked left axis deviation.
    Left ventricular hypertrophy.
(2) Tricuspid atresia.

Discussion

The ECG shows a sinus rhythm with a rate of 115/min. The most obvious abnormality is the presence of huge P waves, indicating marked right atrial hypertrophy. P wave duration is 0.1 s, at the upper limit of normal, and there is terminal P wave inversion in V1. This suggests that left atrial hypertrophy is also present. The P–R interval is normal at 0.16 s. The QRS axis is approximately −70°; there is therefore marked left axis deviation (i.e. the axis is 'superior'). There is also posterior deviation on the horizontal axis, with an abnormal R/S progression. The deep S wave in V3 is due to left ventricular hypertrophy.

This combination of right, or combined, atrial hypertrophy, a superior axis and left ventricular hypertrophy is characteristically found with tricuspid atresia. Other causes of a superior axis in childhood include ostium primum atrial septal defect and severe left ventricular hypertrophy.

Further reading

HARRIS, L. C. and FEINSTEIN, E. (1979) *Understanding ECGs in Infants and Children,* 2nd edn. Boston: Little, Brown and Company

PARK, M. K. and GUNTHEROTH, W. G. (1981) *How to Read Pediatric ECGs.* Chicago: Year Book Medical Publishers Inc.

Answer 121

(1) Cushing's syndrome secondary to adrenal carcinoma.
(2) ACTH levels.
   Abdominal ultrasound.
   Iodocholesterol scintigraphy.
   Renal arteriography.
   CT scan of abdomen.
   Lysine-8-vasopressin test.
(3) Adrenalectomy.

Discussion

This boy is obese without being tall, hypertensive, and has signs of abnormal masculinization for his age. He is polycythaemic and endocrine studies show raised levels of urinary 17-keto- and 17-hydroxysteroids. He has no significant cortisol diurnal variation.

In children, increased secretion from the adrenals is most likely to be due to a malignant tumour of the cortex, benign adenomas being rare. Both are more common in girls (M:F, 1:3). Apart from cortisol there is often increased secretion of adrenal androgens, oestrogens and aldosterone. Abnormal masculinization is common. Growth is usually impaired, although if there is marked virilization it may be normal or even increased. The majority of cases of Cushing's syndrome occur in children under the age of 7, while Cushing's disease (bilateral hyperplasia of the adrenals), although less common, usually occurs in an older age group. The commonest cause of Cushing's syndrome is, however, exogenous steroid therapy.

Investigations commonly show polycythaemia and eosinophilia. Corticosteroids in blood and urine are raised. The cortisol circadian rhythm is lost (normal response 24:00 level >50% 09:00 level). In normal children 0.5 mg dexamethasone 6-hourly will cause serum cortisol suppression. A higher dose of 2 mg 6-hourly causes suppression in adrenal hyperplasia but not in Cushing's syndrome due to adrenal cortical tumours. This test is not always reliable. A very high level of 17-ketosteroids, as seen in this boy, is suggestive of adrenal carcinoma.

Plasma ACTH levels are invariably low or undetectable in adrenal tumours and in autonomous dysplasia (normal values 10–80 pg/ml at 09:00 and <10 pg/ml at midnight). Ultrasound imaging can accurately detect tumours as small as 3–5 cm, and is therefore an important investigation. In iodocholesterol scintigraphy, a tracer dose of cholesterol is injected intravenously, and the abdomen scanned daily from day 4. Best images are usually obtained on day 7. Carcinomas have a low uptake of cholesterol and the adrenals are either poorly visualized or not seen.

Renal arteriography is useful pre-operatively, and may also detect hepatic secondaries. In the lysine-8-vasopressin test, ACTH is measured at 15 and 60 min after an intravenous injection of lysine-8-vasopressin. In adrenal carcinoma levels of ACTH remain low. This test is primarily used for differentiating between pituitary adenomas, where there is an explosive response, and ectopic ACTH with no response.

Treatment consists of adrenalectomy. Unfortunately adrenal carcinomas frequently metastasize to liver and lungs and the prognosis is poor.

Further reading

FOREST, M. G. (1981) Adrenal steroid excess. In *Clinical Paediatric Endocrinology*, edited by C. G. D. Brook, pp. 429–452. Oxford: Blackwell Scientific Publications

PRITCHARD, J. and CRAFT, A. W. (1984) Malignant disease. In *Chemical Pathology in the Sick Child*, edited by B. E. Clayton and J. M. Round, p. 520. Oxford: Blackwell Scientific Publications

Answer 122

(1) Preclinical rickets.
(2) Wrist X-ray.
(3) Vitamin D supplementation.

Discussion

The pre-term infant is at risk of developing rickets because the growth rate may exceed supplies of calcium and vitamin D. Any infant with obstructive jaundice or impaired hepatic function is similarly at risk – remember the growth velocity in the first 6 months of life is at a maximum.

The classical clinical signs of rickets seen in a toddler do not appear in the young infant, as the signs are a reflection of weight bearing on malleable bones (e.g. leg bowing, kyphoscoliosis, pelvic deformity). A rachitic rosary due to flaring of the rib ends may be visible in a thin infant and craniotabes may be palpable.

An X-ray of the wrist will confirm the biochemical suspicion – demonstrating the metabolic effects, namely of fraying, cupping and splaying of the metaphysis.

Management depends on ensuring adequate daily vitamin supply – 3000 IU of vitamin D orally for 4–6 weeks is therapeutic. Where compliance is a potential problem a massive single dose of 300 000 IU has been used – but this runs the risk of inducing vitamin D toxicity. Serial calcium/phosphorus and alkaline phosphatase measurements should be used to monitor the effects of therapy.

Further reading

FORFAR, pp. 166, 1299
NELSON, p. 1655

Answer 123

(1) Epileptiform EEG.
    Macrocytic anaemia.
(2) Folate deficiency due to anticonvulsant medication.

Discussion

The EEG shows characteristic spike waves clearly distinguishable from background activity, as seen in an epileptic convulsion.

The haematological indices show a low haemoglobin, a low red blood cell count and a raised mean cell volume; the anaemia is therefore macrocytic. The white blood cell count and platelet count are also low as is often the case in megaloblastic anaemia. The most likely cause in this boy is folate deficiency secondary to anticonvulsant therapy with either phenytoin, phenobarbitone or primidone. The mechanism is thought to be due to folate malabsorption and/or increased folate metabolism in the liver. The diagnosis should be confirmed by measuring serum and red cell folate and serum vitamin B_{12}.

There is a rare congenital defect described of folate malabsorption combined with an inability to transfer folate from the plasma to the CNS. This is associated with a megaloblastic anaemia, epilepsy, mental retardation and cerebral calcification.

Other anti-folate drugs include oral contraceptives, ethanol, dihydrofolate reductase inhibitors (methotrexate, trimethoprim, pyrimethamine), and those that reduce absorption (sulphasalazine, cholestyramine).

Further reading

CHANARIN, I. (1983) Megaloblastic anaemias. *Medicine International*, **1**, 1185–1189
FORFAR, pp. 683–690

Answer 124

(1) Riley–Day syndrome.
(2) Histamine skin test.
    Methacholine corneal test.
(3) Poor.

Discussion

Riley–Day syndrome is also known as familial dysautonomia.
   While other causes of failure to thrive, recurrent infection and of peripheral neuropathy should be considered, they rarely occur together. A cardinal feature here is lack of tears, and corneal anaesthesia.
   Riley–Day syndrome is an autosomal recessive disorder commonly found in Ashkenazi Jews where the carrier rate is as high as 1%.
   Small unmyelinated fibres are affected mainly – hence the autonomic, pain and temperature indifference, which may lead as in this case to asymptomatic rib fractures.
   Dopamine breakdown products are generally increased (urinary homovanillic acid) while urinary vanillyl mandelic acid (from noradrenaline) is decreased.
   The histamine test (0.04 µg/kg given subcutaneously) normally causes pain and erythema followed by central wheal surrounded by a flare. The pain is less and there is no flare in familial dysautonomia.
   Five per cent methacholine instilled into the corneal sac produces miosis, but does not affect the normal pupil.
   The prognosis is extremely poor with death in childhood from respiratory infections or the effects of hyperpyrexia and dehydration which normally require prompt and rigorous treatment.

Further reading

BRETT, E. M. (Ed.) (1983) *Paediatric Neurology*, p. 116. Edinburgh: Churchill Livingstone
NELSON, p. 1598

Answer 125

(1) A bleed into the psoas muscle.
(2) Abdominal ultrasound.
(3) 30–40% of normal for several days.

Discussion

A haemarthrosis involving the hip joint is unusual in haemophilia – the bleeding generally occurs into 'hinge' joints, i.e. knees, ankles and elbows. The pain in the hip is from movement of the psoas muscle.

The diagnosis can often be made on clinical grounds, but ultrasound is useful if pain prohibits clinical examination.

Management must be very active as large volumes of blood can accumulate in the psoas muscle.

Plasma volume is approximately 50% of blood volume, i.e. 45 ml/kg. A dose of 20 units/kg will therefore achieve levels of 40% (plasma normally contains 1 unit per 1 ml of factor VIII).

Further reading

FORFAR, p. 973
NELSON, p. 1244

Answer 126

(1) Leucoerythroblastic anaemia – 'leukaemoid reaction'.
(2) Pneumonia.
(3) Myeloid leukaemia.
 Myelofibrosis.
 Hodgkin's disease.
 Tuberculosis.
 Intoxication.
 Marrow infiltration.
 Severe haemorrhage or haemolysis.

Discussion

The child can produce a dramatic response to infection – if the white cell count is greater than $40 \times 10^9/l$ then it is termed 'leukaemoid'.

Unlike chronic myelocytic leukaemia, the cells have elevated levels of alkaline phosphatase, show toxic granulation and Döhle's inclusion bodies.

Management is of the underlying disorder, but occasionally a bone marrow examination is required to differentiate the various causes.

Further reading

NELSON, p. 1239

Answer 127

Seven to eight years.

Discussion

Most 'developmental' questions in paediatric membership consist of a written description of a child's behaviour. Increasingly, as community child health is included in basic paediatric training, so more 'developmental' questions will occur.

This test of drawing is included in the Ruth Griffiths Scales of Mental Development in the eighth year, i.e. the child is 7 years old.

The Goodenough Draw a Man test can be used as a very quick 'screen' of hand–eye coordination and cognitive development.

The basal age is 3 years and then for each additional four criteria 1 year of age is added.

The first 20 criteria are:

(1) Head present.
(2) Legs present.
(3) Arms present.
(4) Trunk present.
(5) Length of trunk greater than breadth.
(6) Shoulders indicated.
(7) Both arms and legs attached to the trunk.
(8) Arms and legs attached at correct places.
(9) Neck present.
(10) Neck continuous with head or trunk.
(11) Eyes present.
(12) Nose present.
(13) Mouth present.
(14) Both nose and mouth in two dimensions.
(15) Nostrils indicated.
(16) Hair shown.
(17) Hair non-transparent on more than periphery.
(18) Clothing present.
(19) Two articles of clothing non-transparent.
(20) Entire drawing 'coloured in'.

Answer 128

(1) C3/IgA nephritis (Berger's disease), hydronephrosis or chronic pyelonephritis.
(2) Family history of deafness and nephritis (suggestive of Alport's syndrome).
(3) Renal tract ultrasound or IVU and serum IgA levels.

Discussion

The likely cause of asymptomatic haematuria in this child is either a structural anomaly of the renal tract with or without chronic pyelonephritis, or C3/IgA nephropathy. Other nephritides are unlikely with this history and investigation.

In C3/IgA nephropathy, C3 is deposited in glomerular mesangium but the serum concentration is normal. The serum IgA level, however, is two to three times normal in more than 50% of cases.

Renal tract ultrasound excludes the majority of structural abnormalities, but an IVU is more definitive. Both would also exclude any neoplastic growth, e.g. Wilms' tumour which can occasionally present at this age.

Answer 129

Congenital adrenal hyperplasia, 11β-hydroxylase deficiency.

Discussion

11β-Hydroxylase deficiency is the second most common defect after 21-hydroxylase deficiency causing congenital adrenal hyperplasia. This enzyme is essential for synthesis of both aldosterone and cortisol. There is an increase in both serum 11-deoxycortisol and 11-deoxycortisone. The latter is a precursor of aldosterone, and a mineralocorticoid in its own right. Its accumulation results in hypertension and hypernatraemia (rather than salt depletion as is found in 21-hydroxylase deficiency). Virilization of girls and macrogenitosomia in boys is present from birth. If untreated, progressive hypertension leads to renal failure in later childhood or adulthood.

Further reading

BROOK, C. G. D. (Ed.) (1981) Congenital adrenal hyperplasia. In *Clinical Paediatric Endocrinology*, pp. 453–464. Oxford: Blackwell Scientific Publications

DILLON, M. J. (1981) Salt-losing states. In *Clinical Paediatric Endocrinology*, edited by C. G. D. Brook, pp. 465–478. Oxford: Blackwell Scientific Publications

Answer 130

(1) Right atrial hypertrophy.
    Superior QRS axis.
    Right ventricular hypertrophy.
(2) Complete atrioventricular septal defect.

Discussion

This ECG shows a sinus rhythm, with a rate of 150/min.

P wave duration is normal, but the P wave amplitude (3 mm in II) is increased. Right atrial hypertrophy is therefore present. The P–R interval is 0.12 s (upper limit of normal 0.14 s). The QRS duration is 0.06 s (upper limit of normal 0.06 s) and the QRS axis is approximately −80° (i.e. 'superior'). The QRS voltages are abnormally large, over the right ventricle (VI deflection, 31 mm). Right ventricular hypertrophy is therefore present. The T wave axis is normal (approximately +45°).

These ECG findings are characteristic of a complete atrioventricular septal defect, where in addition to an ostium primum atrial septal defect there is a ventricular septal defect and an atrioventricular valve common to both ventricles. This defect is particularly common in children with Down's syndrome.

Further reading

HARRIS, L. C. and FEINSTEIN, E. (1979) *Understanding ECGs in Infants and Children,* 2nd edn. Boston: Little, Brown and Company

PARK, M. K. and GUNTHEROTH, W. G. (1981) *How to Read Pediatric ECGs.* Chicago: Year Book Medical Publishers Inc.

Answer 131

(1) Restrictive pattern.
(2) Post-radiation therapy fibrosis.

Discussion

This pattern of lung function tests is rare in childhood, but lung function tests are based on physiological principles and therefore most answers can be deduced.

There is usually a primary pathology and the effects on the lungs are secondary.

Any process leading to long-term oedema/inflammation can proceed on to a diffuse pulmonary fibrosis. In broad groups the conditions are as follows:

(1) Alveolar exudates
    renal failure
    cardiac failure
    drug reactions.
(2) Granulomatous processes
    sarcoid
    extrinsic allergic alveolitis.
(3) Inorganic dusts – asbestos etc.
(4) Unknown aetiology, e.g. cryptogenic fibrosing alveolitis.
(5) Post-radiation therapy.

This child's lungs would have been irradiated at the time of spinocranial irradiation during induction therapy for acute lymphoblastic leukaemia. It is likely that this child may also be shorter than expected due to poor spinal growth – a complication not now seen due to intrathecal methotrexate superseding spinal irradiation.

Answer 132

(1) 34.5 kg.
(2) Cerebral gigantism – Sotos syndrome.

Discussion

The answer usually expected is cerebral gigantism, i.e. Sotos syndrome, because in this condition the child is born large and an accelerated growth rate that continues for the first 4–5 years of life is seen.

Biochemically these children are often normal – the presumption being that this is a hypothalamic disorder. They are often slightly dysmorphic with hypertelorism and an antimongoloid slant to the eyes. The hands, feet and jaw are large and there is an excess of subcutaneous tissue – suggesting growth hormone excess – but on testing these are normal.

Other causes of gigantism should be considered, although often these children are normal sized at birth, e.g. pituitary gigantism, Prader–Willi, Beckwith, untreated congenital adrenal hyperplasia and some forms of lipodystrophy.

Further reading

NELSON, p. 1442

Answer 133

(1) Bartter's syndrome.
(2) Sodium replacement.
 Potassium supplements.
 Prostaglandin inhibitors, e.g. indomethacin.
 Renin blockers, e.g. propranolol.
 Blockade of distal tubular potassium secretion, e.g. amiloride.
 Aldosterone antagonists, e.g. spironolactone.

Discussion

Questions on Bartter's syndrome are common in both the long and short cases – it presents in many ways and is not often considered in a list of differential diagnoses.

The exact cause has not been established but the pertinent features are:

(1) Juxtaglomerular apparatus hypertrophy.
(2) Increased renin levels.
(3) Hyperaldosteronism.
(4) Hypokalaemic alkalosis.
(5) Normal blood pressure and no oedema.
(6) Increased prostaglandin E_2 in urine.

Symptomatically, the child may present with reduced growth velocity, weakness, anorexia, salt craving, polydipsia, polyuria, constipation and tetany. Where hypokalaemic alkalosis and normotension coexist without an obvious explanation, think of Bartter's syndrome. A high bicarbonate may be the key to certain questions and so the following may be helpful (the conditions are not listed in order of frequency!):

Metabolic alkalosis with volume expansion
 (1) High BP, high aldosterone, high renin:
   renal artery stenosis
   renin-producing tumour.
 (2) High BP, high aldosterone, low renin:
   primary hyperaldosteronism
   adrenal carcinoma.
 (3) High BP, low aldosterone, low renin:
   DOCA/steroid therapy
   liquorice
   pseudohyperaldosteronism.

Metabolic alkalosis with volume contraction – blood pressure may be low or normal, aldosterone high, renin high:
 vomiting/laxatives (pyloric stenosis)
 cystinosis
 diuretics
 cystic fibrosis
 Bartter's syndrome
 chloride losing enteropathy.

Excess bicarbonate loads
 milk alkali syndrome
 respiratory acidosis.

Contraction alkalosis, e.g. post-nephrotic syndrome diuresis.

Further reading

FORFAR, p. 1024
NELSON, pp. 247, 1490

Answer 134

(1) Type 2 ventilatory failure.
(2) Compensated respiratory acidosis.
(3) Pickwickian syndrome.
(4) Rapid weight reduction.

Discussion

This child is grossly overweight and this had led to hypoventilation from poor chest wall expansion with a reduction in vital capacity and tidal volume. The aterial gases therefore show a low Po_2 and a high Pco_2, i.e. type 2 ventilatory failure. The respiratory acidosis is compensated by a high bicarbonate – not given in the data but inferred by a normal pH in the presence of a high Pco_2. With time, chronic hypoventilation leads to polycythaemia, pulmonary hypertension and cardiac failure.

Rapid weight loss is the treatment of choice. Oxygen therapy is contraindicated as this child relies on oxygen drive to maintain ventilation. Occasionally, respiratory stimulants are required in the short term until weight loss is established.

Further reading

NELSON, p. 170

Answer 135

(1) Ten per cent.
(2) Preconceptual vitamin supplementation.
   Serum α-fetoprotein estimation around 16 weeks gestation.
   Amniocentesis.
   Fetal ultrasound scan.

Discussion

Spina bifida is one of the genetic disorders attributed to a multifactorial inheritance pattern. It occurs in about 2.5 per 1000 live births. The risks to future siblings are about 4% when one child is affected and 10% when two children have been affected. These figures are roughly true for other conditions which are multifactorial, e.g. ventricular septal defects, cleft lip and palate, and congenital dislocation of the hip. It is assumed that a number of minor gene defects (not serious in themselves) occur together, and these, combined with some environmental conditions, cause the defect.

Serum α-fetoprotein should be performed at about 16 weeks. Amniocentesis would be required if this were raised, and may be thought necessary in any event in a woman with this past history. Fetal ultrasound can often show neural tube defects and evidence of hydrocephaly. Trials have shown that preconceptual vitamin supplementation has had beneficial effects in preventing the recurrence of these abnormalities. Usually one tablet of Pregnavite Forte F is taken three times a day for one month prior to conception.

Further reading

FORFAR, p. 693

Answer 136

(1) Renal vein thrombosis.
(2) Obstructive nephropathy.
 Acute tubular necrosis.
 Renal trauma with perirenal haematoma.
 Bacterial or fungal infection.
 Unilateral cystic kidney.
 Nephroblastoma.
 Neuroblastoma.
(3) Urea and electrolytes, clotting studies, abdominal ultrasound.
(4) Glucose tolerance test.

Discussion

Possible causes of a unilaterally enlarged kidney in the neonatal period are listed above. If one assumes the first day examination excluded the presence of significant enlargement, then this has developed since birth. Although there are several possible diagnoses that should be kept in mind, the most likely cause in this baby who is ill is a renal vein thrombosis.

The majority of infants (75%) with renal vein thrombosis present during the first month of life (30% in the first week, 45% in the first month). In the neonatal period it is commoner in boys than girls (ratio 2:1). In approximately 50% the thrombosis is bilateral. Usually it occurs during severe illness, though rarely there may be no obvious cause. There is often a history of diarrhoea preceding the anuria/haematuria. Hypertension is not usually present. If the condition is not detected early, a metabolic acidosis ensues and this may present with respiratory distress or tachypnoea.

Affected kidneys are usually papable. An ultrasound examination will also confirm an enlarged kidney and may also show renal vein occlusion. These infants sometimes require peritoneal dialysis – a decision based primarily on the creatinine and electrolyte findings. There is often a degree of disseminated intravascular coagulation. Clotting studies are indicated before correction with fresh frozen plasma.

This is a large infant who required a lower segment caesarean section. There is an increased incidence of renal vein thrombosis in infants of diabetic mothers and a maternal glucose tolerance test should be performed.

Further reading

FORFAR, p. 1072
NELSON, p. 397

Answer 137

(1) Infantile cortical hyperostosis (Caffey's disease).
(2) Osteomyelitis of the mandible.
(3) X-ray of mandible.
    Blood cultures.

Discussion

Infantile cortical hyperostosis is a disease of unknown aetiology primarily involving the flat bones – with the mandible, clavicles and the ends of the ulnae being the most commonly affected sites. Initially, there is intraperiosteal inflammation which may extend into the local tissues. This then changes to fibrous tissue which, in turn, is replaced by periosteal new bone. Eventually the process resolves and the affected bones are remodelled to their original contours. While the process is active a pseudoarthrosis may be present.

The presentation has many features in common with osteomyelitis except for the multiple site involvement and, in a child of this age, the distribution of bones affected (osteomyelitits may affect the maxilla, humerus and femur in the neonatal period).

The X-ray shows characteristic signs of infantile cortical hyperostosis – the correct diagnosis depending on this finding.

Further reading

FORFAR, pp. 197, 1606, 1614
NELSON, p. 1650

Answer 138

(1) Physiological.
(2) Wood's light examination.

Discussion

The distribution of the calcification is not mentioned, but in an otherwise normal child the most likely reason is physiological. Structures which may calcify include the choroid plexus (in over 2-year-olds), interclinoid and petroclinoid ligaments, the falx cerebri, the tentorium cerebelli, pacchionian granulations and, later in childhood, the pineal. There is increased likelihood of calcification with age.

The pathological causes in one major series (Willich) included *Toxoplasma* (22%), Sturge–Weber (7.8%), intracranial haemorrhage (7.3%), tumour related (7.2%) and tuberous sclerosis (4%).

Much rarer causes include vascular malformations, neurofibromatosis, pseudohypoparathyroidism, neurofibromatosis, pseudohypoparathyroidism, 'idiopathic functional cerebrovascular ferocalcinosis' and cytomegalovirus infection.

The genetic implications of neurofibromatosis and tuberose sclerosis are important. The Wood's light test is easy to perform and so this is the most important single test.

Providing the child's neurological system is intact, the fundi are clear and the calcification does not appear pathological, there would be no good indication to proceed to a CT scan as an intracranial space-occupying lesion is unlikely

It is worth looking at the fundi for chorioretinitis as the diagnosis of *Toxoplasma* can often be made on ophthalmological examination.

Answer 139

(1) Eisenmenger syndrome with ventricular septal defect.
(2) No.

Discussion

The catheter data show near identical pressures in the pulmonary artery aorta and left and right ventricles. There is a decrease in oxygen saturation from the left atrium to the left ventricle. The findings are those of a large ventricular septal defect with pulmonary hypertension and a right-to-left shunt.

Eisenmenger syndrome refers to any condition where pulmonary vascular hypertension is at or above systemic level and there is a right-to-left or bidirectional shunt at ventricular, atrial, or aortopulmonary level. It occurs when irreversible pulmonary hypertension develops as a consequence of large defects between the systemic and pulmonary circulations and therefore can be a complication of a ventricular septal defect, atrial septal defect, patent ductus arteriosus, aortopulmonary window, or with more complex congenital heart disease.

Once the Eisenmenger syndrome has developed there is no corrective treatment available, either surgical or medical.

Further reading

JORDON, S. C. and SCOTT, O. (1981) *Heart Disease in Paediatrics,* 2nd edn, pp. 274–278. London: Butterworths

Index

Page numbers in italic type refer to the Answers section.

Acidosis, metabolic, 5, *82*
Abetalipoproteinaemia, 6, *85*
ABO incompatibility and neonatal jaundice, 63, *166*
Abscess, cerebral, 10–11, *93*
Addison's disease, 3, *79–80*
Adrenal disorders,
    carcinoma and Cushing's syndrome, 65, *168–169*
    hyperplasia, congenital, 70, *174*
    in neonate, 16, *99*
Agammaglobulinaemia, X-linked, 51, *149–150*
Aldosteronism, *see* Hyperaldosteronism, secondary
Alveolar capillary block, 16, *100*
Ampicillin rash and mononucleosis, 53, *152–153*
Amylo-1,6-glucosidase deficiency, *159*
Amyloid and juvenile arthritis, *108*
Anaemias, 37, *128*
    and Crohn's disease, 9, *90*
    haemolytic, 17–18, *101–102*
        autoimmune, 44, *139–140*
        and hereditary spherocytosis, 6, *84*
        and iron deficiency, 61, *163*
    leucoerythroblastic, from pneumonia, 69, *172*
    macrotic, and epilepsy, 67, 68, *170*
    sideroblastic, hereditary, *128*
Angioneurotic oedema, hereditary, 38–39, *129–130*
Antidiuretic hormone secretion, inappropriate, 8, *88*
α,-Antitrypsin deficiency and neonatal jaundice, 31, *120–121*
Aortic coarction and Turner's syndrome, 54, *155*
Apnoea, neonatal, hypoglycaemic, 64, *167*

Arteriovenous fistula, post-traumatic, 59, *160*
Arthritis, chronic juvenile,
    and anaemia, *128*
    Type I pauciarticular, 24, *108–109*
Asphyxia at birth and hyperinsulinism, 46, *142–143*
Asthma 23, *107–108*
Ataxias, 52, *151–152*
    telangiectasia, 61–62, *164*
Atrial disorders,
    atrioventricular septal defect, and Down's syndrome, 70–72, *174–175*
    fibrillation, 49, *145–146*
    flutter, 39, *131*
    left atrial hypertrophy, 24–25, *109–110*
    septal defect, ostium secundum, 13–14, *94–95*
Autosomal recessive inheritance, 46, *143*

Bartter's syndrome, 72, *176–177*
Bacterial infection and chronic granulomatous disease, *116*
Berger's disease, 70, *173–174*
Biliary atresia, neonatal, 15, *97–98*
Bilirubin and neonatal jaundice, 7, *86–87*
    conjugated hyperbilirubinaemia, 15, *97–98*
Bleeding,
    and Glanzman's disease, 12, *93*
    and infectious mononucleosis, 53, *152–153*
    in premature noenate, 50–51, *148–149*
    in von Willebrand's disease, 6, *83*

Blood,
  haemarthrosis and haemophilia, 69, 171–172
  haematuria, 70, 173–174
  haemoglobinuria and sulphasalazine-related haemolysis, 39, 130
  incompatibility and neonatal jaundice,
    ABO, 63, 166
    rhesus, 63, 134, 166
  platelets in von Willebrand's disease, 83
  see also Anaemias: Bleeding; Bruising; Haemolytic disorders; Haemophilia: Leukaemia
Bodian-Shwachman syndrome, 3, 5, 81
Bone transplantation for granulomatous disease, 116
  see also Marrow hypoplasia
Breast feeding,
  and infant jaundice, 86
  milk composition, 109
  passing maternal blood, 27–28, 115
Bruising and Glanzman's disease, 12, 93
Bruton's disease, 51, 149–150

Caffey's disease, 74–75, 180
Calcification, intracerebral, 75, 181
  see also Hypercalcaemia, idiopathic
Candidiasis syndrome in Addison's disease, 80
Carcinoma, adrenal, and Cushing's syndrome, 65, 168–169
  see also Tumours
Cardiomyopathy, congestive, 60, 161
  see also Heart disorders
Cerebral disorders,
  abscess, 10–11, 93
  ataxia, cerebellar, 52, 151–152
  calcification, intracerebral, 75, 181
  encephalitis, herpes simplex, 45, 141–142
  gigantism, 72, 73, 176
  hydrocephalus and meningomyelocele, 74, 178
Cerebellar ataxia, 52, 151–152
Chemotherapy and renal failure, 15, 96
Chickenpox and cerebellar ataxia, 151–152
Chloridorrhea, congenital, in neonate, 18, 103
Clinitest positive for urine, 15, 96–97

Congenital adrenal hyperplasia, 70, 174
  in neonate, 16, 99
Conjunctivae,
  bulbar, telangiectasia of, 61–62, 164
  icteric, and spherocytosis, 6
Convulsions,
  and anti-diuretic hormone secretion, 8, 88
  and glycogen storage disease, 58, 158–159
  'grand mal', haemolytic uraemic syndrome, 56, 155–156
  and hypoglycaemia, neonatal, 64, 167
  and ornithine carbamoyl transferase deficiency, 53–54, 153
  'petit mal' absences, 63, 166
  see also Infantile spasms
Copper deficiency and anaemia, 128
Cortical hyperostosis, infantile, 74–75, 180
Crohn's disease, 9, 90
Cushing's syndrome and adrenal carcinoma, 65, 168–169
Cystic fibrosis, 57, 157–158
  complications, 63, 165–166
  and nasal polyposis, 34, 36, 125
Cystinosis and Franconi's syndrome, 132–133
Cystinuria and renal colic, 22, 105–106

Deafness, see Hearing loss
Diabetes,
  DIDMOAD syndrome, 40, 131–132
  insipidus, in Wolfram syndrome, 40, 131–132
  and ketoacidosis, 49, 146–147
  maternal, and neonatal hypoglycaemia, 46, 142–143
  mellitus, 25, 110–111
    and dwarfism, 30, 118
    and hypothyroidism, 30, 118
    in Wolfram syndrome, 40, 131–132
  Somogyi effect in, 44, 139
Diarrhoea and vomiting,
  and hypernatraemic dehydration, 32, 122
  and hyponatraemic dehydration, 17, 100–101
DIDMOAD syndrome, 40, 131–132
Diethyltriamine pentaacetic acid renogram, 47, 145
Down's syndrome,
  atrioventricular septal defect in, 70–72, 174–175
  inheritance risk, 31, 119–120

Drug overdose and cerebellar ataxia, 52, *151–152*
Dubin–Johnson syndrome, *126*
Duodenal ulcer, 26, *112*
Dwarfism,
  diabetic, 30, *118*
  and growth hormone deficiency, *104*
Dysplasia, polyostotic fibrous, 33–34, *123–124*

Ear typanograms, middle-ear fluid *vs* drum perforation, 58, *159*
  see also Eustachian tube blockage; Hearing loss
Ebstein's anomaly and Wolff–Parkinson–White syndrome, 79
Eczema and Wiskott–Aldrich syndrome, 10, 92
Edward's syndrome, 38, *129*
Eisenmenger syndrome and ventricular septal defect, 75, *181–182*
Emphysema and α_1-antitrypsin deficiency, *121*
Encephalitis, herpes simplex, 45, *141–142*
Encephalopathy, lead, 22, *106–107*
Enteropathy, protein losing, 58–59, *160*
Epilepsy,
  poor control of, 44, *140*
  therapy and macrocytic anaemia, 67, 68, *170*
  see also Convulsions; Infantile spasms
Epistaxia in Glanzman's disease, 12, *93*
Eustachian tube blockage, 42, *135–136*
Eyes, *see* Optical disorders

Fibrosis, post-radiation therapy, 72, *175–176*
Fisher's syndrome, 152
Franconi's syndrome, 40, *132–133*
Fungal infection and granulomatous disease, *116*

Galactosaemia in neonate, 45, *141*
Gigantism, cerebral, 72, 73, *176*
Glanzman's disease, 12, *93*
Glucose-6-phosphate dehydrogenase deficiency,
  and glycogen storage disease, *158–159*
  and heredity, 43, *138*
  and neonatal haemolysis, *134*

Glycogen storage disease, 58, *158–159*
Goodenough Draw a Man Test, 33, 69, *123, 173*
Granulomatous disease, chronic, 28, *115–116*
Growth,
  delay, transient, 92
  hormone deficiency, 92
  isolated, 20–21, *104–105*
Guillain-Barré syndrome, 52, *150–151*

Haemarthrosis in haemophilia, 69, *171–172*
Haematuria, 70, *173–174*
Haemoglobinuria and sulphasalazine-related haemolysis, 39, *130*
Haemolytic disorders,
  anaemia, 17–18, *101–102*
  in cystic fibrosis, 57, *157–158*
  uraemic syndrome, 56, *155–156*
Haemophilia,
  bleed into psoas muscle, 69, *171–172*
  vs. von Willebrand's disease, 83
Hand abnormality and Edward's syndrome, *129*
Hashimoto's disease and Turner's syndrome, 34, *124–125*
Hearing loss,
  high frequency, 36–37, *126*
  from otitis media, 12, *94*
  in Wolfram's syndrome, 40, *131–132*
Heart disorders,
  aortic coarction and Turner's syndrome, 54, *155*
  block, third degree, 43, *138–139*
  cardiomyopathy, congestive, 60, *161*
  congenital, in neonate, 56, *156–157*
  failure,
    congestive, 60, *161*
    right, in cystic fibrosis, 63, *165–166*
  mitral valve prolapse and Wolff–Parkinson–White syndrome, 79
  right bundle branch block after heart surgery, 18, 19, *102–103*
  see also Atrial disorders; Ventricular disorders
Helminth infection, Toxocara, 57, *157*
Hepatitis,
  giant cell, and α_1-antitrypsin, deficiency, *120*
  neonatal, 15, *97–98*
  from Rubella, *vs.* galactosaemia, 45, *141*

Herpes simplex encephalitis, 45, *141–142*
Hydrocephalus and meningomyelocele, 74, *178*
Hydronephrosis, 47, 70, *145, 173–174*
11β-Hydroxylase deficiency, 70, *174*
Hyparrhythmia, 47, 48, *144–145*
Hyperaldosteronism, secondary,
  and chloridorrhea, 103
  and renovascular hypertension, 8–9, *89*
Hyperbilirubinaemia, conjugated, in neonatal jaundice, 15, *97–98*
Hypercalcaemia, idiopathic, 37, *127*
Hyperinsulinism, neonatal, 46, *142–143*
Hypernatraemic dehydration, 32, *122*
Hyperostosis, cortical, infantile, 75–76, *180*
Hyperoxia in premature neonate, 50–51, *148–149*
Hypoalbuminaemia in protein losing enteropathy, 58–59, *160*
Hypoglycaemia, neonatal, 46, *142–143*
  and apnoea, 64, *167*
Hyponatraemic dehydration, 17, *100–101*
Hypotension and lactic acidosis, 5, *82*
Hypothyroidism and diabetes mellitus, 30, *118*
Hysteria and respiratory alkalosis, 42–43, *137*

Ileal disease, Crohn's disease as, *90*
Immerslund–Grasbeck syndrome and vitamin B_{12}, *90*
Immunological abnormalities in Wiskott–Aldrich syndrome, 10, *92*
Inappropriate antidiuretic hormone syndrome, 8, *88*
Infant feeding, milks compared, 24, *109*
  see also Breast feeding
Infantile spasms, 47, 48, *144–145*
Insulin, *see* Hyperinsulinism, neonatal
Intussusception, surgery for, and antidiuretic hormone secretion, 8, *88*
Iridocyclitis, chronic, and juvenile arthritis, *108*
Iron deficiency anaemia, 61, *163*

Jaundice,
  and autoimmune haemolytic anaemia, 44, *139–140*
  neonatal, 63, *166*
    and α_1-antitrypsin deficiency, 31, *120–121*
  and breast milk, 7, *86–87*
  haemolytic, 41, *134–135*
  and hepatitis, 45, *141*
  and hepatitis/biliary atresia, 15, *97–98*
  and spherocytosis, *84*
  and Rotor syndrome, 36, *125–126*

Ketoacidosis, diabetic, 49, *146, 147*
Kidney, *see* Adrenal disorders; Renal disorders
Klinefelter's syndrome, 23, *107*

Lactic acidosis, 5, *82*
Laryngeal oedema and angioneurotic oedema, *129*
Lead poisoning, 22, 2106–107
  and anaemia, *128*
Left atrial hypertrophy, 24–25, *109–110*
Left ventricular hypertrophy, 28–29, *117*
Leucoerythroblastic anaemia from pneumonia, 69, *172*
Leukaemia,
  lymphoblastic, chemotherapy and renal failure, 15, *96*
  and pleural effusion, 28, *116–117*
  and pneumonia, 69, *172*
Lipoproteinaemia, 6, *85*
Liver biopsy, neonatal, in hepatitis/biliary atresia, *98*
  see also Hepatitis
Lung function,
  and alveolar capillary block, 16, *100*
  and myasthenia gravis, juvenile,, 40–41, *133*
  see also Pulmonary disorders; Pleural effusion; Pleurisy; Respiratory disorders

McCune–Albright syndrome, 33–34, *123–124*
Macrotic anaemia and epilepsy, 67, 68, *170*
Marrow hypoplasia, 26, *112–113*
Mauriac's syndrome, 30, *118*

Meningitis,
  bacterial, partially treated, 62, *165*
  tuberculous, 16, *98*
Meningomyelocele and hydrocephalous, 74, *178*
Mental development and drawing tests, 33, 42, 59, *123*, *136–137*, *173*
  Denver Developmental Screening Test, 50, *148*
Metabolic acidosis in neonate, 56, *156–157*
Milk compositions for infant feeding, 24, *109*
  see also Breast feeding
Mitral valve prolapse and Wolff–Parkinson–White syndrome, *79*
Mononucleosis, infectious, 53, *152–153*
Myasthenia gravis, juvenile, 40–41, *133*

Nephritis, C3/IgA, 70, *173–174*
Nephrotic syndrome, neonatal, 25–26, *111*
Nose bleed and infectious mononucleosis, 53, *152–153*

Obesity and Pickwickian syndrome, 73–74, *178*
Optical disorders,
  damage and juvenile arthritis, *108*
  acuity, and Toxacara infection, 57, *157*
  atrophy in Wolfram syndrome, 40, *131–132*
  see also Conjunctivae
Ornithine carbamoyl transferase deficiency, 53–54, *153*
Otitis media, 12, *94*
  and agammaglobulinaemia, 51, *149–150*
Ovarian tumour, oestrogen-secreting, 27, *113*
Oxygen therapy for pre-term infant, 22, *106*

Pancreatic deficiency and Bodian–Shwachman syndrome, 3, 5, *81*
'Petit mal' absences, 63, *166*

Phenobarbitone overdose, 52, *151–152*
Phenytoin overdose, 52, *151–152*
Pickwickian syndrome, 73–74, *178*
Pigmentation in Addison's disease, *79–80*
Pineal tumour, 60, *161–162*
Platelets in von Willebrand's disease, *83*
Pleural effusion, 28, *116–117*
Pleurisy, *116–117*
Pneumonia,
  and agammaglobulinaemia, 51, *149–150*
  and leukaemoid reaction, 69, *172*
Pneumothorax and asthma, 23, *107–108*
Poliomyelitis, *151*
Polydipsia,
  in distal renal acidosis, 50, *147–148*
  psychogenic, 13, *95*
Polymyositis, 151
Polyneuritis, post-infectious, and respiratory failure, 61, *162–163*
Polyostotic fibrous dysplasia, 33–34, *123–124*
Polyposis, nasal, and cystic fibrosis, 34, 36, *125*
Polyuria in distal renal acidosis, 50, *147–148*
Protein losing enteropathy, 58–59, *160*
Puberty, precocious,
  female,
    and ovarian tumour, oestrogen-secreting, 27, *113*
    and polyostotic fibrous dysplasia, 33–34, *123–124*
  male, and pineal tumour, 60, *161–162*
Pulmonary disorders,
  alveolar capillary block, 16, *100*
  arteriovenous fistula, post-traumatic, 59, *160*
  hypertension in cystic fibrosis, 63, *165–166*
  pneumonia,
    and agammaglobulinaemia, 51, *149–150*
    and leukaemoid reaction, 69, *172*
  pneumothorax and aminophylline suppository, 23, *107–108*
  see also Respiratory disorders
Pyelonephritis, chronic, 70, *173–174*
Pyruvate kinase deficiency and neonatal haemolysis, *134*

Renal disorders,
  colic and cystinuria, 22, *105–106*
  failure,
    and leukaemia chemotherapy, 15, *96*
    and haemolytic uraemic syndrome, *156*
    and rickets, 41, *135*
  hydronephrosis, 47, 70, *145, 173–174*
  nephritis, C3/IgA, 70, *173–174*
  nephrotic syndrome, neonatal, 25–26, *111*
  tubular acidosis,
    distal, 50, *147–148*
    proximal, primary, 30, *118–119*
  renal vein thrombosis in neonate, 74, *179–180*
Renovascular hypertension and secondary hyperaldosteronism, 8–9, *89*
Respiratory disorders,
  acidosis, compensated, in cystic fibrosis, 34, 36, *125*
  alkalosis and hysteria, 42–43, *137*
  distress in premature neonate, 50–51, *148–149*
  and oxygen therapy, 22, *106*
  failure, type II, and polyneuritis, 61, *162–163*
Rhesus incompatibility and neonatal jaundice, 63, *134, 166*
Rickets, 41, *81, 135*
  and Fanconi's syndrome, 40, *132–133*
  preclinical, in premature neonate, 65, 67, *169–170*
Right bundle branch block after heart surgery, 18, 19, *102–103*
Riley-Day syndrome, 67, *171*
Rose bengal excretion and biliary atresia, 97
Rotor syndrome, 36, *125–126*
Rubella infection in neonate, 45, *141*
Ruth Griffiths Scales of Mental Development, 33, 69, *123, 173*

Salicylate poisoning, 27, *114*
Septicaemia and lactic acidosis, 5, *82*
Sick cell syndrome, *146–147*
Sickle cell β⁰-thalassaemia and splenomegaly, 31, *121–122*
Sideroblastic anaemia, hereditary, *128*
Sodium, *see* Hypernatraemic dehydration; Hyponatraemic dehydration
Somogyi effect in diabetes, 44, *139*

Sotos syndrome, 72, 73, *176*
Spherocytosis, hereditary, 6, *84*
Spina bifida and meningomyelocele, 74, *178*
Spinal cord tumour, *151*
Spleen,
  and sickle cell β⁰-thalassaemia, 31, *121–122*
  in spherocytosis, hereditary, 6, *84*
Squint and tuberculous meningitis, 16
Stature,
  and Crohn's disease, 9, *20*
  and growth hormone deficiency, isolated, 20–21, *104–105*
  and transient growth delay, 10, *92*
  and Turner's syndrome, 34, *124–125*
  see also Dwarfism; Gigantism
Steatorrhoea, 6, *85*
Streptococcal, group B, disease in neonate, 56, *156–157*
Stridor and hypocalcaemic tetany, 5, *81*
Supraventricular tachycardia, 54, 55, *154*

Telangiectasia, ataxia, 61–62, *164*
Tetany, hypocalcaemic, 5, *81*
Thalassaemia,
  and anaemia, *128*
  vs. iron deficiency anaemias, *163*
  and neonatal haemolysis, *134*
Thyroiditis, lymphocytic, and Turner's syndrome, 34, *124–125*
  see also Hypothyroidism and diabetes mellitus
Toxins, environmental, and marrow hypoplasia, 26, *112–113*
Toxocara infection, 57, *157*
Tricuspid atresia, 65, 66, *167–168*
Trisomy-18, 38, *129*
Tuberculosis and pleural effusion, 28, *116–117*
Tumours, 11, *93*
  lysis syndrome and renal failure, 15, *96*
  ovarian, oestrogen-secreting, 27, *113*
  pineal, 60, *161–162*
  spinal cord, *151*
Turner's disease, 9, *61*
Turner's syndrome, 54, *155*
  and lymphocytic thyroiditis, 34, *124–125*
Tympanograms, 58, *135–136, 159*

Ulcer, duodenal, 26, *112*
Uraemic syndrome, 56, *155–156*
Urea cycle disorders, 53–54, *153*

Ventricular disorders,
  extrasystoles, 35, *124*
  left ventricular hypertrophy, 28–29, *117*
  septal defect, 7, *87–88*
    and Eisenmenger syndrome, 75, *181–182*
  supraventricular tachycardia, 54, 55, *154*
Vitamins,
  B$_{12}$, absorption in Crohn's disease, *90*
  D,
    deficiency and hypocalcaemic tetany, *81*
    and idiopathic hypercalcaemia, *127*
    for pre-clinical rickets, *169–170*

Vitamins (*cont.*)
  E,
    and abetalipoproteinaemia, *85*
    deficiency and cystic fibrosis, 57, *157–158*
von Gierke's disease, *158*
von Willebrand's disease, 6, *83*

Weidemann–Beckwith syndrome and neonatal hyperinsulinism, 46, *142–143*
Wiskott–Aldrich syndrome, 10, *92*
Wolff–Parkinson–White syndrome, 4, *79*
  and atrial fibrillation, *146*
Wolfram syndrome, 40, *131–132*

Zollinger–Ellison syndrome, *112*